WHO guidelines

WHO guidelines for screening and treatment of precancerous lesions for cervical cancer prevention

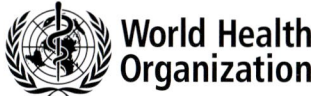

WHO Library Cataloguing-in-Publication Data

WHO guidelines for screening and treatment of precancerous lesions for cervical cancer prevention.

I.World Health Organization.

ISBN 978 92 4 154869 4
Subject headings are available from WHO institutional repository

© World Health Organization 2013

All rights reserved. Publications of the World Health Organization are available on the WHO web site (www.who.int) or can be purchased from WHO Press, World Health Organization, 20 Avenue Appia, 1211 Geneva 27, Switzerland (tel.: +41 22 791 3264; fax: +41 22 791 4857; e-mail: bookorders@who.int).

Requests for permission to reproduce or translate WHO publications –whether for sale or for non-commercial distribution– should be addressed to WHO Press through the WHO web site (www.who.int/about/licensing/copyright_form/en/index.html).

The designations employed and the presentation of the material in this publication do not imply the expression of any opinion whatsoever on the part of the World Health Organization concerning the legal status of any country, territory, city or area or of its authorities, or concerning the delimitation of its frontiers or boundaries. Dotted lines on maps represent approximate border lines for which there may not yet be full agreement.

The mention of specific companies or of certain manufacturers' products does not imply that they are endorsed or recommended by the World Health Organization in preference to others of a similar nature that are not mentioned. Errors and omissions excepted, the names of proprietary products are distinguished by initial capital letters.

All reasonable precautions have been taken by the World Health Organization to verify the information contained in this publication. However, the published material is being distributed without warranty of any kind, either expressed or implied. The responsibility for the interpretation and use of the material lies with the reader. In no event shall the World Health Organization be liable for damages arising from its use.

Printed in Spain

Contents

Lists of participants	v
Process for managing declarations and conflicts of interest	ix
Acknowledgements	x
Acronyms and abbreviations	xi
Executive summary	xii
Screen-and-treat strategy summary recommendations	xiv
1. Introduction	1
Target audience	2
Purpose	2
2. Methods	4
Guideline groups	4
Formulating questions and determining outcomes	4
Synthesis of the evidence and preparation of evidence profiles	5
Modelling of health outcomes	6
Development of the recommendations	7
Guideline review and approval process	8
3. Recommendations	9
Important considerations that apply to all screen-and-treat recommendations	9
Screen-and-treat recommendations	10
4. Research gaps and further considerations	16
5. Use of the guideline	18
Guideline dissemination	18
Guideline evaluation	18
Guideline update	19
References	20

Annexes

Annex 1: Declarations of Interest	22
Annex 2: Decision-making flowchart for screen-and-treat strategies	25
Annex 3: Flowcharts for screen-and-treat strategies (negative or unknown HIV status)	26
Screen with an HPV test and treat with cryotherapy or LEEP	26
Screen with an HPV test followed by VIA and treat with cryotherapy or LEEP	27
Screen with VIA and treat with cryotherapy or LEEP	28
Screen with an HPV test followed by colposcopy (with or without biopsy) and treat with cryotherapy or LEEP	29
Screen with cytology followed by colposcopy (with or without biopsy) and treat with cryotherapy or LEEP	30
Annex 4: Flowcharts for screen-and-treat strategies (HIV-positive status or unknown HIV status in areas with high endemic HIV infection)	31
Screen with an HPV test and treat with cryotherapy or LEEP	31
Screen with an HPV test followed by VIA and treat with cryotherapy or LEEP	32
Screen with VIA and treat with cryotherapy or LEEP	33
Screen with an HPV test followed by colposcopy (with or without biopsy) and treat with cryotherapy or LEEP	34
Screen with cytology followed by colposcopy (with or without biopsy) and treat with cryotherapy or LEEP	35
Annex 5: Search strategies for evidence reviews	36
Annex 6: PRISMA flow diagram for inclusion and exclusion of studies for evidence reviews	38
Annex 7: Reference list of all studies included in the evidence reviews	39

Supplemental material*: GRADE evidence-to-recommendation tables and evidence profiles for each recommendation

    Section A. Negative or unknown HIV status

    Section B. HIV-positive status or unknown HIV status in areas with high endemic HIV infection

---

* Available online: www.who.int/reproductivehealth/publications/cancers/screening_and_treatment_of_precancerous_lesions/en/index.html

Lists of participants

WHO Steering Group

Nathalie Broutet (lead)
Reproductive Health and Research
WHO Headquarters

Jean-Marie Dangou
Disease Prevention and Control
WHO Regional Office for Africa

Ibtihal Fadhil
Noncommunicable Diseases
WHO Regional Office for the Eastern Mediterranean

Gunta Lazdane
Sexual and Reproductive Health
WHO Regional Office for Europe

Silvana Luciani
Cancer Prevention and Control
WHO Regional Office for the Americas /
Pan American Health Organization (PAHO)

Arvind Mathur
Making Pregnancy Safer and Reproductive Health
WHO Regional Office for South-East Asia

Amolo Okero
Counselling and Testing, HIV/AIDS
WHO Headquarters

Somchai Peerapakorn
Reproductive Health
WHO Country Office – Thailand

Andreas Ullrich
Chronic Diseases Prevention and Management
WHO Headquarters

Cherian Varghese
Noncommunicable Diseases and Health Promotion
WHO Regional Office for the Western Pacific

Adriana Velazquez
Essential Medicines and Pharmaceutical Policies
WHO Headquarters

Marco Vitoria
HIV Treatment and Care
WHO Headquarters

Lawrence Von Karsa
Quality Assurance and Screening
International Agency for Research on Cancer

Guideline Development Group

Marc Arbyn
Unit of Cancer Epidemiology
Scientific Institute of Public Health – Louis Pasteur
Brussels, Belgium

Paul D. Blumenthal
Population Services International (PSI)
Stanford University School of Medicine
Department of Obstetrics and Gynecology
Stanford, USA

Joanna Cain (Chair)
Portland, USA

Michael Chirenje
Department Obstetrics and Gynaecology
University of Zimbabwe Medical School
Harare, Zimbabwe

Lynette Denny
Department Obstetrics and Gynaecology
Groote Schuur Hospital
Cape Town, South Africa

Hugo De Vuyst
Infections and Cancer Epidemiology
International Agency for Research on Cancer
Lyon, France

Linda O'Neal Eckert
Department of Global Health
Gynecology Director
Harborview Center for Sexual Assault and
Traumatic Stress
Seattle, USA

Sara Forhan
HIV Care and Treatment Branch
Global AIDS Program
Centers for Disease Control and Prevention (CDC)
Atlanta, USA

Eduardo Franco
Division of Cancer Epidemiology
McGill University
Montreal QC, Canada

Julia C. Gage
Division of Cancer Epidemiology and Genetics
National Cancer Institute
Rockville, USA

Francisco Garcia
American Cancer Society
Tucson, USA

Rolando Herrero
Prevention and Implementation Group
International Agency for Research on Cancer
Lyon, France

José Jeronimo
PATH
Seattle, USA

Enriquito R. Lu
Jhpiego
Baltimore, USA

Silvana Luciani
Cancer Prevention and Control
PAHO
Washington DC, USA

Swee Chong Quek
Women's and Children's Hospital
Singapore

Rengaswamy Sankaranarayanan
Prevention and Implementation Group
International Agency for Research on Cancer
Lyon, France

Vivien Tsu
PATH
Seattle, USA

Methods Group

Based at MacGRADE Collaborating Centre,
McMaster University, Hamilton, Canada:
systematic review team and GRADE
methodologists

Holger Schünemann (Lead Investigator)
Department of Clinical Epidemiology and
Biostatistics

Reem A. Mustafa (Coordinator)
Department of Clinical Epidemiology and
Biostatistics

Nancy Santesso (Coordinator)
Department of Clinical Epidemiology and
Biostatistics

External Review Group

Irene Agurto
Santiago, Chile

Ahti Anttila
Mass Screening Registry
Finnish Cancer Registry
Helsinki, Finland

Partha Sarathi Basu
Department of Gynecologic Oncology
Chittaranjan National Cancer Institute
Kolkata, India

John-Paul Bogers
Laboratorium voor Cel – en Weefselleer
Faculteit Geneeskunde
Campus Groenenborger
Antwerp, Belgium

August Burns
Grounds for Health
Waterbury, USA

Rolando Camacho-Rodriguez
Cancer Control Coordinator
Programme of Action for Cancer Therapy
International Atomic Energy Agency
Vienna, Austria

Silvia de Sanjosé
Institut Català d'Oncologia
L'Hospitalet de Llobregat
Barcelona, Spain

Anne Garnier
Department of Cancer Screening
Institut National du Cancer (INCa)
Boulogne-Billancourt, France

Martha Jacob
Kochi
Kerala State, India

Namory Keita
Department of Gynecology and Obstetrics
Donka Teaching Hospital
Conakry, Republic of Guinea

Nancy Kidula
ACCESS Uzima, Jhpiego
Nairobi, Kenya

Rajshree Jha Kumar
Mumbai, India

Anne Levin
Bethesda, USA

Khunying Kobchitt Limpaphayom
Department of Obstetrics and Gynecology
Faculty of Medicine
Chulalongkorn University
Bangkok, Thailand

Ian Magrath
International Network for Cancer Treatment and Research
Brussels, Belgium

Raul Murillo
Subdireccion Investigaciones y Salud Pública
Instituto Nacional de Cancerología de Colombia
Bogotá, Colombia

Daniel Murokora
Uganda Women's Health Initiative
Kampala, Uganda

Oneko Olola
Kilimanjaro Christian Medical Centre
Moshi, Tanzania

Groesbeck Parham
Centre for Infectious Disease Research in Zambia
Lusaka, Zambia

Patrick Petignant
Surgical Gynecologic Oncology Unit
Hôpital Cantonal
Geneva, Switzerland

Ilka Rondinelli
International Planned Parenthood Federation
London, United Kingdom

Carlos Santos
Instituto Nacional de Enfermedades Neoplásicas
Lima, Peru

Mona Saraiya
Division of Cancer Prevention and Control
National Center for Chronic Disease Prevention and Health
CDC
Atlanta, USA

Achim Schneider
Klinik für Gynäkologie und Gynäkologische
Onkologie
CharitéCentrum
Berlin, Germany

Nereo Segnan
Department of Cancer Screening
and Unit of Cancer Epidemiology
Piemonte and San Giovanni University
Hospital
Turin, Italy

Tshewang Tamang
Vaccine Preventable Disease Program
Ministry of Health
Thimphu, Bhutan

Nguyen-Toan Tran
Geneva, Switzerland

Jérôme Viguier
Santé Publique
INCa
Boulogne-Billancourt, France

Steven Weyers
Department of Obstetrics and Gynecology
Ghent University Hospital
Gent, Belgium

Katherine Worsley
Marie Stopes International
London, United Kingdom

Eduardo Zubizarreta
International Atomic Energy Agency
Vienna, Austria

Process for managing declarations and conflicts of interest

Roles of the technical and working groups

In September 2010, the External Review Group (ERG) met to decide on the update of *Comprehensive cervical cancer control: a guide to essential practice* (C4-GEP), which was originally published in 2006. One of the major conclusions was that the chapter on screening and treatment of precancerous lesions for cervical cancer prevention needed to be updated. This group also made recommendations to the World Health Organization (WHO) on the composition of the Guideline Development Group (GDG).

In 2011, the GDG and the Methods Group (MG) met several times in joint sessions to develop the PICO questions (population, intervention, comparison, outcome), to select and rate the importance of the outcomes for treatment of precancerous cervical lesions and for the screen-and-treat approach to prevent cervical cancer, and to discuss and agree on the methodology and the key parameters to be considered in the modelling exercise to evaluate the outcomes of the screen-and-treat algorithm.

In April 2012, the GDG, the MG and the ERG met in a joint session to discuss the results of the literature review and the outcomes of the modelling exercise, and to prepare the draft recommendations.

In 2012 and 2013, the GDG and the MG met several times in joint sessions, either by conference call or in person, to further discuss and finalize the draft recommendations. These draft recommendations were then sent to the ERG for endorsement.

Management of conflicts of interest

Conflicts of interest were managed as follows:

1. All experts who participated in the process were required to complete the WHO Declaration of Interest (DOI) form before they commenced their work for WHO, and to promptly notify WHO if any change in the disclosed information occurred during the course of this work. The completed DOI forms were reviewed by the WHO Secretariat with a view to managing disclosed interests in the field of cervical cancer screening and treatment.

2. At the meeting of the ERG in September 2010 and at the first joint meeting of the GDG, MG and the ERG in 2013, each expert disclosed his/her declared interests to the other experts as part of the round of introductions at the beginning of the meeting so that the group was aware of any existing interests among the members.

3. All declared interests have been reviewed by WHO's Office of the Legal Counsel. The decision was that all experts could participate in the process but interests should be disclosed in the guideline.

4. All relevant declared interests (15 out of 54 experts) are summarized in this report (see Annex 1).

It should be noted that these guidelines focus on cervical screening to detect precancerous lesions in order to allow early treatment and thus prevent these from evolving into cancerous lesions. These guidelines do not address primary prevention of cervical cancer through vaccination against human papillomavirus (HPV).

Acknowledgements

The World Health Organization (WHO) would like to thank the members of the Guideline Development Group and the Methodology Group for their constant availability and hard work. WHO is also very grateful to the External Review Group for making possible the development of these essential recommendations for screening and treatment of precancerous lesions for cervical cancer prevention. The names of the participants in each group are listed on pages v–viii.

In addition, we would like to thank the following staff, fellows, and students from McMaster University, Hamilton, Canada, who contributed to the work of the systematic review but were not included in the discussion on recommendations: Adrienne Cheung, Charmaine Fraser, Shreyas Gandhi, Jessica Hopkins, Rohan Kehar, Rasha Khatib, Nancy Lloyd, Ahmad Mustafa, Marco Perez, and Wojtek Wiercioch.

WHO also wishes to express sincere gratitude to the Flanders International Cooperation Agency (FICA), the Institut National du Cancer (INCa), France, and the GAVI Alliance (formerly the Global Alliance for Vaccines and Immunisation) for providing the main funding for this document.

Editing, proofreading, design and layout: Green Ink (greenink.co.uk)

Acronyms and abbreviations

ASCUS	atypical squamous cells of undetermined significance
CIN	cervical intraepithelial neoplasia
CKC	cold knife conization
ERG	External Review Group
FICA	Flanders International Cooperation Agency
GAVI Alliance	formerly the Global Alliance for Vaccines and Immunisation
GDG	Guideline Development Group
GRADE	Grading of Recommendations, Assessment, Development and Evaluation
HPV	human papillomavirus
IARC	International Agency for Research on Cancer
INCa	Institut National du Cancer (France)
LEEP	loop electrosurgical excision procedure (also LLETZ)
LLETZ	large loop excision of the transformation zone (also LEEP)
MG	Methods Group
NCI	National Cancer Institute (USA)
NIH	National Institutes of Health (USA)
PAHO	Pan American Health Organization
Pap test	Papanicolaou test (cytology-based method for cervical cancer screening)
PICO	population, intervention, comparison, outcome
PRISMA	Preferred Reporting Items for Systematic Reviews and Meta-Analyses
QUADAS	QUality Assessment for Diagnostic Accuracy Studies
VIA	visual inspection with acetic acid
WHO	World Health Organization

Executive summary

Cervical intraepithelial neoplasia (CIN) is a premalignant lesion that may exist at any one of three stages: CIN1, CIN2, or CIN3. If left untreated, CIN2 or CIN3 (collectively referred to as CIN2+) can progress to cervical cancer. Instead of screening and diagnosis by the standard sequence of cytology, colposcopy, biopsy, and histological confirmation of CIN, an alternative method is to use a 'screen-and-treat' approach in which the treatment decision is based on a screening test and treatment is provided soon or, ideally, immediately after a positive screening test. Available screening tests include a human papillomavirus (HPV) test, visual inspection with acetic acid (VIA), and cytology (Pap test). Available treatments include cryotherapy, large loop excision of the transformation zone (LEEP/LLETZ), and cold knife conization (CKC).

This guideline provides recommendations for strategies for a screen-and-treat programme. It builds upon the existing *WHO guidelines: Use of cryotherapy for cervical intraepithelial neoplasia* (published in 2011) and on the new *WHO guidelines for treatment of cervical intraepithelial neoplasia 2–3 and glandular adenocarcinoma in situ* (being published concomitantly with these present guidelines). This guideline is intended primarily for policy-makers, managers, programme officers, and other professionals in the health sector who have responsibility for choosing strategies for cervical cancer prevention, at country, regional and district levels.

For countries where a cervical cancer prevention and control programme already exists, these recommendations were developed to assist decision-makers to determine whether to provide a different screening test followed by a different treatment, or to provide a series of tests followed by an adequate treatment. For countries where such a programme does not currently exist, these recommendations can be used to determine which screening test and treatment to provide. In addition to the recommendations, a decision-making flowchart is also proposed in Annex 2 to help programme managers choose the right strategy based on the specific country or regional context. Once the strategy has been chosen, the appropriate screen-and-treat flowchart for that strategy can be followed. The flowcharts for all strategies are provided in Annex 3 (specifically for women of negative or unknown HIV status), and Annex 4 (for women of HIV-positive status or unknown HIV status in areas with high endemic HIV infection).

The methods used to develop these guidelines follow the *WHO handbook for guideline development*, and are described in Chapter 2 of this document. A Guideline Development Group (GDG) was established that included experts, clinicians, researchers in cervical cancer prevention and treatment, health programme directors and methodologists. Conflicts of interest were managed according to World Health Organization (WHO) rules. An independent group of scientists at a WHO collaborating centre conducted systematic reviews on the diagnostic accuracy of the available screening tests and the effects of different treatments for CIN (see Annexes 5–7). This evidence was used to model and compare different screen-and-treat strategies in women of unknown HIV status and women of HIV-positive and HIV-negative status and the results were presented to the GDG in evidence tables following the GRADE (Grading of Recommendations, Assessment, Development and Evaluation) approach. The GRADE evidence profiles and evidence-to-recommendation tables for each recommendation are available online (Supplemental material, Sections A and B).

This guideline provides nine recommendations for screen-and-treat strategies to prevent cervical cancer. While a brief summary of the recommendations is included on the next page, the complete recommendations with remarks and a summary of the evidence for each are found in Chapter 3 of this document.

Although the best evidence to assess the effects of a screen-and-treat strategy is from randomized controlled trials, we identified few randomized controlled trials that evaluated these strategies and reported on patient-important outcomes. Areas for future research include screen-and-treat strategies using a sequence of tests (e.g. HPV test followed by VIA); screen-and-treat strategies in women of HIV-positive status; and measurement of important health outcomes following a screen-and-treat strategy.

Screen-and-treat strategy summary recommendations

These recommendations apply to all women regardless of HIV status, but specific recommendations for women living with HIV have been developed.

> **The expert panel[1] recommends** against the use of CKC as a treatment in a screen-and-treat strategy. Therefore, all screen-and-treat strategies below involve treatment with cryotherapy, or LEEP when the patient is not eligible for cryotherapy.
>
> **The expert panel suggests:**
>
> ▸ Use a strategy of screen with an HPV test and treat, over a strategy of screen with VIA and treat. In resource-constrained settings, where screening with an HPV test is not feasible, the panel suggests a strategy of screen with VIA and treat.
>
> ▸ Use a strategy of screen with an HPV test and treat, over a strategy of screen with cytology followed by colposcopy (with or without biopsy) and treat. However, in countries where an appropriate/high-quality screening strategy with cytology followed by colposcopy already exists, either an HPV test or cytology followed by colposcopy could be used.
>
> ▸ Use a strategy of screen with VIA and treat, over a strategy of screen with cytology followed by colposcopy (with or without biopsy) and treat. The recommendation for VIA over cytology followed by colposcopy can be applied in countries that are currently considering either programme or countries that currently have both programmes available.
>
> ▸ Use a strategy of screen with an HPV test and treat, over a strategy of screen with an HPV test followed by colposcopy (with or without biopsy) and treat.
>
> ▸ Use either a strategy of screen with an HPV test followed by VIA and treat, or a strategy of screen with an HPV test and treat.
>
> ▸ Use a strategy of screen with an HPV test followed by VIA and treat, over a strategy of screen with VIA and treat.
>
> ▸ Use a strategy of screen with an HPV test followed by VIA and treat, over a strategy of screen with cytology followed by colposcopy (with or without biopsy) and treat.
>
> ▸ Use a strategy of screen with an HPV test followed by VIA and treat, over a strategy of screen with an HPV test followed by colposcopy (with or without biopsy) and treat.

---

[1] The expert panel includes all members of the WHO Steering Group, the Guideline Development Group (GDG), and the External Review Group (ERG).

As shown below, a decision-making flowchart has been developed that will assist programme managers to choose one of the suggested strategies, depending on the context where it will be implemented (also provided in Annex 2). Details about the flow of each different strategy are also presented in the flowcharts in Annex 3 (for women of negative or unknown HIV status) and Annex 4 (for women of HIV-positive status or unknown HIV status in areas with high endemic HIV infection).

Decision-making flowchart for programme managers

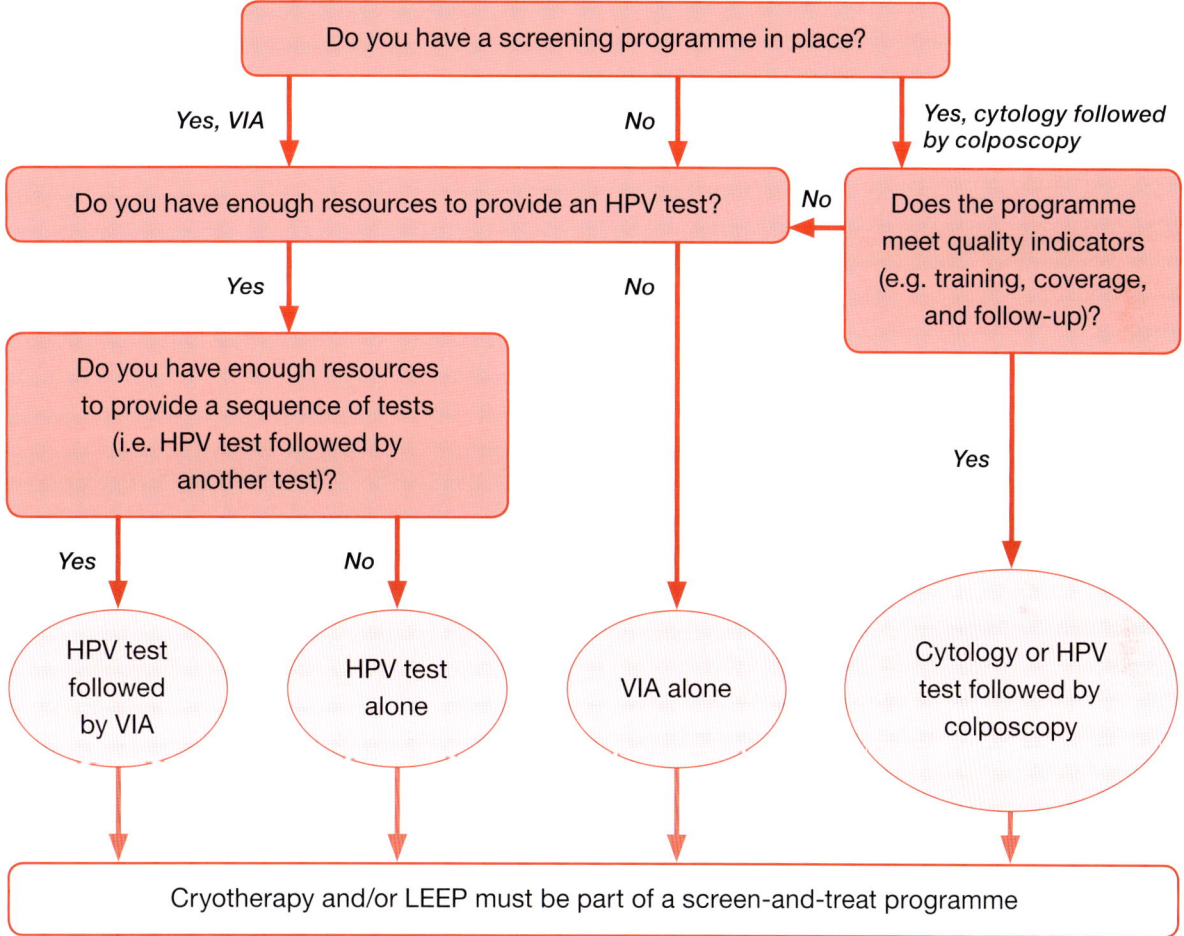

Note: each light-pink bubble refers to one strategy in Annex 3 (for women of negative or unknown HIV status) or Annex 4 (for women of HIV-positive status or unknown HIV status in areas with high endemic HIV infection).

1. Introduction

Cervical intraepithelial neoplasia (CIN) is a premalignant lesion that may exist at any one of three stages: CIN1, CIN2, or CIN3.[2] If left untreated, CIN2 or CIN3 (collectively referred to as CIN2+) can progress to cervical cancer. It is estimated that approximately 1–2% of women have CIN2+ each year. This rate is reported to be higher in women of HIV-positive status, at 10% *(1–5)*. The standard practice is to screen women using cytology (Pap test), and when cytology results are positive the diagnosis of CIN is based on subsequent colposcopy, biopsy of suspicious lesions, and then treatment only when CIN2+ has been histologically confirmed. This traditional screening method requires highly trained human resources and a substantial amount of laboratory equipment. In low- and middle-income countries, because of the high cost of setting up screening programmes based on cytology, coverage of screening is very low and alternative screening methods are needed. In addition, follow-up of a positive cytology test with colposcopy and biopsy requires resources and skilled personnel that are largely lacking in many countries. Other bottlenecks in screening programmes based on cytology include the need for referral to distant health facilities for diagnostic and treatment services, and the long waiting times before cytology results are available. An alternative approach to diagnosing and treating CIN is to use a 'screen-and-treat' approach in which the treatment decision is based on a screening test, and not on a histologically confirmed diagnosis of CIN2+, and treatment is provided soon or, ideally, immediately after a positive screening test.

The goal of a screen-and-treat programme for cervical cancer is to reduce cervical cancer and related mortality with relatively few adverse events. The programme must include a screening test or strategy (sequence of tests) and be linked to appropriate treatments for CIN, and also provide referral for treatment of women with invasive cervical cancer. Common screening tests that are widely used include tests for human papillomavirus (HPV), cytology (Pap test), and unaided visual inspection with acetic acid (VIA). These tests can be used as a single test or in a sequence. When using a single test, a positive result indicates the need for treatment. When using a sequence of tests, women who test positive on the first test receive another test and only those who test positive on the second test are treated. Women with a positive first screening test followed by a negative second screening test are followed up. Available treatments include cryotherapy, large loop excision of the transformation zone (LEEP/LLETZ), and cold knife conization (CKC).

This guideline provides recommendations for strategies for a screen-and-treat programme. It builds upon the existing recommendations for the use of cryotherapy to treat CIN *(6, 7)* and on the new *WHO guidelines for treatment of cervical intraepithelial neoplasia 2–3 and glandular adenocarcinoma in situ (8)*, which is being published concomitantly with these present guidelines. When developing the guideline, the Guideline Development Group (GDG) considered that countries currently providing screen-and-treat programmes may be uncertain about which strategy to use. Therefore, these recommendations were developed by comparing the benefits and harms of different screen-and-treat strategies. For countries where a cervical cancer prevention and control programme already exists, these recommendations were developed to assist decision-makers to determine whether to provide a different screening test

---

[2] Diagnosis of CIN is established by histopathological examination of a cervical punch biopsy or excision specimen. A judgement of whether or not a cervical tissue specimen reveals CIN, and to what degree, is dependent on the histological features concerned with differentiation, maturation and stratification of cells and nuclear abnormalities. The proportion of the thickness of the epithelium showing mature and differentiated cells is used for grading CIN. More severe degrees of CIN are likely to have a greater proportion of the thickness of epithelium composed of undifferentiated cells, with only a narrow layer of mature differentiated cells on the surface *(9)*.

followed by a different treatment instead, or to provide a series of tests followed by an adequate treatment. For countries where such a programme does not currently exist, these recommendations can be used to determine which screening test and treatment to provide. In addition, a decision-making framework is proposed in Annex 2 to help programme managers choose the right strategy based on the specific country or regional context.

The recommendations and background information about the various screening tests and treatments are also available in an updated version of *Comprehensive cervical cancer control: a guide to essential practice* (C4-GEP) *(10)*. The C4-GEP was originally published in 2006 by the World Health Organization (WHO) to assist clinicians and programme managers to diagnose and treat CIN in order to prevent and control cervical cancer. In 2009, WHO committed to updating the C4-GEP as specific aspects deserved the development of new recommendations. In particular, new evidence had become available regarding the use of cryotherapy for CIN (a new guideline was completed in 2011 *[7]*); treatment of histologically confirmed CIN2+ (a new guideline is being published concomitantly with this present one *[8]*); and strategies for screening and treatment of precancerous cervical lesions (the subject of this present guidance). In addition, there is a new awareness that when making recommendations for screen-and-treat strategies, the consequences of treating or not treating women after positive or negative screening results should also be considered. Typically, the selection of a screening test is based on its accuracy, which is determined by calculating the sensitivity and specificity of the test, and recommendations are based on that evidence. However, these data, do not address the consequences of screening and treating women. When deciding on a screen-and-treat strategy, it is critical to consider the downstream consequences after treatment (for a positive test) or no treatment (for a negative test), such as cervical cancer and related

mortality, recurrence of CIN2+, adverse effects of treatment (and overtreatment), and use of resources. These recommendations are based on evidence about the diagnostic accuracy of each of the screening tests, together with evidence about the benefits and harms of treatments.

Target audience

This guideline is intended primarily for policy-makers, managers, programme officers, and other professionals in the health sector who have responsibility for choosing strategies for cervical cancer prevention, at country, regional and district levels. Individuals working in reproductive health care programmes, particularly programmes for the prevention of sexually transmitted infections (STIs) including HIV/AIDS and for family planning, at the district and primary health care levels, should also consult these guidelines to understand how recommendations are developed and why it is vitally important to select and implement evidence-based strategies to prevent cervical cancer.

Purpose

This guideline provides recommendations for screen-and-treat strategies to prevent cervical cancer (Chapter 3). In addition to the recommendations, this document proposes a decision-making flowchart for choosing the best screen-and-treat strategy for a particular setting at a programme level (Annex 2); and – for use once the strategy is chosen – the screen-and-treat flowcharts for all strategies are provided, including the flowcharts specifically for women of negative or unknown HIV status (Annex 3), and those for women of HIV-positive status or of unknown HIV status in areas with areas with high endemic HIV infection (Annex 4). This document also describes the WHO methodology that was used for the development of these recommendations (Chapter 2, and Annexes 5–7), and provides GRADE (Grading of

Recommendations, Assessment, Development and Evaluation) evidence profiles[3] and evidence-to-recommendation tables[4] for each recommendation (available online: Supplemental material, Sections A and B). This document provides the scientific background and justification for the practical information found in the C4-GEP *(10)*.

---

[3] The GRADE evidence profiles summarize the evidence from the systematic reviews and the model, as well as the quality of the evidence.

[4] The 'evidence-to-recommendation tables' describe the process of going from the evidence to developing the recommendations, and explain the judgements and rationale for factors that are not part of the GRADE evidence profiles.

2. Methods

The methods used to develop these guidelines followed the *WHO handbook for guideline development (11, 12)*.

Guideline groups

WHO formed a Guideline Development Group (GDG) for the screen-and-treat strategies to prevent cervical cancer, chaired by Joanna Cain. The 17 selected members provided expert clinical guidance and support throughout the guideline development process. WHO also selected an External Review Group (ERG) comprising 33 professionals, including health-care providers with experience in screening and treating CIN, pathologists, researchers in cervical cancer prevention and treatment, programme directors, health educators, epidemiologists, public health officers, nurses and methodologists. A Methods Group (MG) from the MacGRADE Centre at McMaster University, a WHO collaborating centre, provided expertise in evidence synthesis and guideline development processes.

Formulating questions and determining outcomes

In February 2011, the GDG met to discuss the questions and outcomes to address in the chapter on screen-and-treat strategies to appear in the updated C4-GEP, in order to incorporate new evidence. The GDG identified 15 potential questions to guide the evidence review for screening options and treatment strategies for cervical pre-cancer. The MG surveyed the GDG anonymously online using Survey Monkey[5] to prioritize the questions and determine which ones are clinically relevant or used in practice; 14 out of 17 members responded. Among the 15 questions, the GDG identified 7 that related to comparisons between standard screen-and-treat strategies and those that are NOT typically used in practice (e.g. an HPV test followed by cytology), and therefore these seven questions were excluded. The remaining eight questions were retained as the basis for the screening recommendations (see Box 1).

During this same meeting, the GDG developed a list of outcomes that should be considered when making decisions and recommendations for the screen-and-treat strategies. These outcomes were informed by the work previously conducted for the preparation of the WHO guidelines entitled *Use of cryotherapy for cervical intraepithelial neoplasia (7)*. Following the meeting, the MG surveyed all GDG and ERG members online using Survey Monkey to identify and rank the critical outcomes for making recommendations. Participants ranked outcomes on a scale from 1 (not at all important) to 7 (critical) in terms of importance for decision-making. Thirty of the

---

Box 1: Prioritized questions for screening options for cervical pre-cancer

1. Should an HPV test or VIA be used to screen?
2. Should an HPV test or cytology followed by colposcopy (with or without biopsy) be used to screen?
3. Should VIA or cytology followed by colposcopy (with or without biopsy) be used to screen?
4. Should an HPV test or an HPV test followed by colposcopy (with or without biopsy) be used to screen?
5. Should an HPV test followed by VIA or an HPV test as a single test be used to screen?
6. Should an HPV test followed by VIA or VIA as a single test be used to screen?
7. Should an HPV test followed by VIA or cytology followed by colposcopy (with or without biopsy) be used to screen?
8. Should an HPV test followed by VIA or an HPV test followed by colposcopy (with or without biopsy) be used to screen?

---

[5] Survey Monkey: www.surveymonkey.com

50 members surveyed provided responses and an average ranking was calculated for each outcome. Outcomes with an average ranking of 4 (important) or higher were included in the evidence review and considered when making the recommendations (see Box 2).

Synthesis of the evidence and preparation of evidence profiles

A screen-and-treat strategy is made up of two linked parts: the screening test(s) followed by treatment of CIN. The best studies to inform screen-and-treat recommendations are randomized controlled trials in which women are randomized to receive 'screen-and-treat strategy A' or 'screen-and-treat strategy B', and health outcomes of all of the women are measured and presented (even those who had false-negative screening results and were never treated). However, few such studies have been conducted; most studies do not link the screening strategy with the treatment and the outcomes. Instead, there are studies that measure the accuracy of a test to diagnose CIN (without reporting on treatment), and there are other studies that only measure health outcomes of screen-positive women after treatment. Hence, the outcomes for women with true-negative or false-negative screening results are not measured. This is true for the literature for cervical pre-cancer screening; few studies report health outcomes of all women who were screened, including those who were treated and those who were not. For this reason, the primary evidence used to develop these screen-and-treat recommendations could not be based on evidence from randomized controlled studies. Instead, these recommendations are based on modelling health outcomes from a series of reviews of the diagnostic accuracy of the available screening tests, and a series of reviews of the effects of the various treatments for CIN.

The MG searched the MEDLINE and EMBASE online databases up to February 2012 for screening strategies related to an HPV test compared to VIA, and VIA compared to cytology. A separate search was conducted to update a Cochrane Review that was in progress for an HPV test compared to cytology up to November 2012. Another search was conducted for colposcopy up to September 2012 (see Annex 5 for search strategies). The MG used the evidence on treatment of CIN that was concurrently being gathered for the development of *WHO guidelines for treatment of cervical intraepithelial neoplasia 2–3 and glandular adenocarcinoma in situ (8)*. The searches were not restricted by language or study design in order not to exclude primary studies or previously published systematic reviews in this area. Reference lists of relevant studies were reviewed and the WHO GDG was contacted for additional references.[6]

At least two members of the MG independently screened titles and abstracts and the full text of relevant articles, and a third investigator resolved disagreements. The MG included observational studies for diagnostic test accuracy studies considered at low risk of bias. For example, all women in the studies had to receive both screening tests that

> **Box 2: Outcomes for screen-and-treat strategies identified as important for making recommendations (in order of importance)**
>
> 1. Mortality from cervical cancer
> 2. Cervical cancer incidence
> 3. Detected CIN2, CIN3
> 4. Major infections (requiring hospital admission and antibiotics, e.g. pelvic inflammatory disease)
> 5. Maternal bleeding
> 6. Premature delivery
> 7. Fertility
> 8. Identification of STIs (benefit)
> 9. Minor infections (requiring outpatient treatment only)

---

[6] Details of the methods for the systematic reviews are available at the WHO website.

were being compared, and all women who tested positive or negative (or a random sample of at least 10% of the women who tested negative) had to receive the 'gold standard' diagnostic test. Studies had to include non-pregnant women aged 18 years or older who had not been treated previously for CIN. Women could be of HIV-positive or HIV-negative status or of unknown HIV status. The Preferred Reporting Items for Systematic Reviews and Meta-Analyses (PRISMA) checklist was used to develop the flow diagram for inclusion and exclusion of studies (Annex 6). A list of all studies included in the reviews of diagnostic test accuracy is provided in Annex 7.

Two members of the MG independently abstracted data about patient characteristics, setting, and diagnostic test accuracy, using a pre-tested data abstraction form. Data to assess the quality of the studies was also collected with the QUADAS tool (QUality Assessment for Diagnostic Accuracy Studies) *(13)*. We pooled the diagnostic test accuracy data using Stata 12 data analysis and statistical software.

The MG developed a mathematical model to calculate the benefits and harms of each screen-and-treat strategy compared to other screen-and-treat strategies for women of unknown HIV status and for women of HIV-positive status. CIN2+ prevalence, natural progression data, the pooled diagnostic test accuracy results, and pooled data on treatment effects and complications were all considered in the model (see Annex 7 for references used in the model). The estimates of the expected absolute effects on health-care outcomes and a summary of the model assumptions are provided transparently in the evidence profiles for women of negative or unknown HIV status and for women of HIV-positive status (see Supplemental material, Sections A and B, available online) and for women of different ages.

Two members of the MG evaluated the quality of evidence using the Grading of Recommendations Assessment, Development and Evaluation (GRADE) approach *(14, 15)* and presented the evidence and its quality in the GRADE evidence profiles. Evidence for diagnostic accuracy of the screening tests is presented in evidence profiles for diagnostic test accuracy for each recommendation (see Supplemental material, Sections A and B, generally in section 2.1 for each recommendation). The evidence from the model (i.e. outcomes after a screen-and-treat strategy) is also presented in evidence profiles (see Supplemental material, Sections A and B, generally in sections 2.2 and 2.3 for each recommendation, according to age). The quality of the evidence or confidence in the effect estimates was assessed as high ⊕⊕⊕⊕, moderate ⊕⊕⊕⊖, low ⊕⊕⊖⊖, or very low ⊕⊖⊖⊖, according to the GRADE criteria. Tables to facilitate decision-making for recommendations (evidence-to-recommendations tables) were produced for each recommendation. These tables include a summary of the evidence (benefits and harms), an assessment of the quality of the evidence, relevant patient values and preferences, and any implications for use of resources and feasibility (Supplemental material, Sections A and B).

Modelling of health outcomes

A screening test with the highest diagnostic accuracy is not necessarily the test of choice in clinical practice. The decision to recommend a screening test needs to be justified by its impact on downstream patient-important health outcomes. Decision analysis is a powerful tool for evaluating a diagnostic or screening test on the basis of long-term patient-important outcomes when only intermediate outcomes – such as test sensitivity and specificity – are known. When making the decision to recommend a diagnostic or screening test, a panel should consider the health outcomes downstream from the test. For example, the health risks of interventions resulting from false-positive (FP) and false-negative (FN) findings should be compared with the health benefits associated with true-negative (TN) and true-positive (TP) findings.

To inform these recommendations, we built a mathematical model using TreeAge Pro 2012 software. In this model we calculated the proportions of TP, TN, FP and FN findings for each of the screening tests (VIA, HPV and cytology) given the pooled test-accuracy estimates and the pretest probability of having CIN in that population. We then calculated the probability of developing any of the critical outcomes for decision-making (see Box 2) based on the treatment they may receive and the pooled estimates of efficacy and potential complications of the different treatments (cryotherapy, CKC and LEEP). To calculate an overall estimate of the outcome, we added the probability of developing an outcome for each of the categories (TP, TN, FP, FN) for the same screening test and treatment option. We identified our assumptions for the models a priori. These assumptions are summarized in the Supplemental material available online, Sections A and B (below each GRADE evidence table for patient-important outcomes following different screen-and-treat strategies). We also specified a priori the sensitivity analysis we performed based on HIV status (HIV-positive compared to unknown HIV status) and different age categories.

Development of the recommendations

In early 2012 (26–28 April), the GDG, the ERG and the MG met to discuss the recommendations. One member each from the GDG and the MG chaired the meeting, which was attended by experts from around the world, representing various public health and medical disciplines. To expand the geographical representativeness of the GDG, it was decided that the ERG – a large group with members representing many countries – would participate in the development of the recommendations during that meeting. Members of the MG presented evidence profiles and evidence-to-recommendation tables, which included evidence about the benefits and harms, values and preferences, resources and feasibility.

With regard to patient values and preferences, the GDG agreed that the evidence found could be applied across all recommendations *(16–18)*. The evidence from qualitative studies suggests that women may fear screening and may have a high level of anxiety related to colposcopy or treatment, and may feel burdened by the need for a second visit for treatment. However, once women decide to be screened they find the screening tests and immediate treatment acceptable. Evidence from the systematic reviews demonstrated that there is a preference for more frequent screening and active management among women who have screened positive for CIN1. In addition, evidence from controlled trials showed that women find treatment by cryotherapy and LEEP acceptable, and are satisfied with a screen-and-treat approach *(19)*.

WHO has recently developed the *WHO cervical cancer prevention and control costing tool (20)*. This tool includes two modules: one on the cost of HPV vaccination and the other on the cost of a screen-and-treat programme. The purpose of the tool is to help programme managers develop a budget for the programme. In order to develop the tool, the cost of each intervention was collected for a range of countries and the calculation tables were developed. This, in addition to the experience of the members of the ERG, was essential to the discussion of the resources needed for each of strategy.

Recommendations were made by the GDG and ERG by balancing the overall desirable and undesirable consequences of the screen-and-treat strategies, which included consideration of important outcomes, values and preferences, resources and feasibility, along with the level of certainty of that information. Members of the panel made decisions based on consensus and unanimous voting, which was not anonymous. The results of those discussions are documented in the evidence-to-recommendation tables for each recommendation, available online in Supplemental material, Sections A and B. The GDG and ERG also identified key research gaps. All the discussions and decisions took place during the April 2012 meeting and no major discord was noted.

The recommendations were assessed as 'strong' or 'conditional', in accordance with the *WHO handbook for guideline development* (*11, 12*). Strong recommendations have been worded as 'we recommend' and conditional recommendations as 'we suggest'. A strong recommendation means that it was clear to the panel that the net desirable consequences of the specified strategy outweighed those of the alternative strategy. But a conditional recommendation was made when it was less clear whether the net desirable consequences of the specified strategy outweighed those of the other strategy. In this guideline, many recommendations are conditional. Table 1 provides a guide to the interpretation of the strength of the recommendations.

Guideline review and approval process

The WHO screen-and-treat strategies to prevent cervical cancer underwent the following peer review process before and during development:

- The questions formulated for the development of the guidelines were circulated among the WHO Steering Group, who also discussed them with the GDG. When the GDG and the WHO Steering Group had reached agreement on the questions, these were sent to the ERG.
- The protocol for systematic reviews was circulated among the GDG. This protocol was also discussed during the ERG meeting, which was also attended by the European Guidelines Development Group in addition to the WHO Steering Group, the GDG and the MG. During that meeting the evidence that had been identified and the draft evidence profiles were discussed.
- Discussions and conference calls were regularly held with the GDG to discuss the data from the literature review, the models, the estimated parameters to include in the models, and the outcomes.
- The final draft guideline with the recommendations was circulated among the members of the GDG for review before WHO clearance.

Table 1. Interpretation of strong and conditional recommendations

Implications	Strong recommendation "We recommend… "	Conditional recommendation "We suggest… "
For patients	Most individuals in this situation would want the recommended course of action, and only a small proportion would not. Formal decision aids are not likely to be needed to help individuals make decisions consistent with their values and preferences.	The majority of individuals in this situation would want the suggested course of action, but many would not.
For clinicians	Most individuals should receive the intervention. Adherence to this recommendation according to the guideline could be used as a quality criterion or performance indicator.	Clinicians should recognize that different choices will be appropriate for each individual and that clinicians must help each individual arrive at a management decision consistent with his or her values and preferences. Decision aids may be useful to help individuals make decisions consistent with their values and preferences.
For policy-makers	The recommendation can be adopted as policy in most situations.	Policy-making will require substantial debate and involvement of various stakeholders.

3. Recommendations

To aid decision-making by programme managers, a decision-making flowchart or algorithm is provided for choosing the best screen-and-treat strategy for a particular setting at a programme level (see Annex 2). Once the strategy has been chosen, flowcharts for each strategy can be followed; these are provided in Annex 3 (negative or unknown HIV status) and Annex 4 (HIV-positive status or unknown HIV status in areas with high endemic HIV infection). The algorithm and the flowcharts are based on the recommendations detailed in this chapter.

Important considerations that apply to all screen-and-treat recommendations

Population targeted by the recommendations

The recommendations in this guideline apply to women 30 years of age (recommended age to start screening) and older because of their higher risk of cervical cancer. However, the magnitude of the net benefit will differ among age groups and may extend to younger and older women depending on their baseline risk of CIN2+. Priority should be given to screening women aged 30–49 years, rather than maximizing the number of screening tests in a woman's lifetime. Screening even once in a lifetime would be beneficial. Screening intervals may depend on financial, infrastructural, and other resources.

For women of HIV-positive status, or of unknown HIV status in areas with high endemic HIV infection, the following should be noted. Although the evidence about screening and treatment to prevent cervical cancer is of lower quality for women who are HIV-positive than for women who are HIV-negative or of unknown HIV status, cervical cancer screening should be done in sexually active girls and women, as soon as a woman or a girl has tested positive for HIV.

Supplemental material, Section A (negative or unknown HIV status) and Section B (HIV-positive status or unknown HIV status in areas with high endemic HIV infection) provide the evidence and judgements for each recommendation (this material is available online).

Considerations for screening tests

The recommendations include strategies based on three screening tests: HPV (cut-off level ≥1.0 pg/ml), cytology (cut-off level ASCUS+, atypical squamous cells of undetermined significance), and VIA. VIA is appropriate to use in women whose transformation zone is visible (typically in those younger than 50). This is because once menopause occurs, the transformation zone, where most precancerous lesions occur, frequently recedes into the endocervical canal and prevents it from being fully visible.

Considerations for treatments

For all screen-and-treat recommendations, cryotherapy is the first-choice treatment for women who have screened positive and are eligible for cryotherapy. When women have been assessed as not eligible for cryotherapy, LEEP is the alternative treatment. Eligibility for cryotherapy follows the guidance provided in the update of the C4-GEP *(10)*: Screen-positive women are eligible for cryotherapy if the entire lesion is visible, the squamocolumnar junction is visible, and the lesion does not cover more than 75% of the ectocervix. If the lesion extends beyond the cryoprobe being used, or into the endocervical canal, the patient is not eligible for cryotherapy and LEEP is the alternative option.

Before treatment, ALL women who have screened positive with any test (but especially with an HPV test) should be visually inspected with acetic acid to determine eligibility for cryotherapy and to rule out large lesions or suspected cervical cancer. VIA should be performed by a trained provider.

Note that there is a distinction in these recommendations between (a) using VIA to determine eligibility for treatment (i.e. cryotherapy versus LEEP), and (b) using VIA as a screening test to determine whether or not to treat.

a. In the 'HPV test' screen-and-treat strategy, women who are HPV-negative are not treated. Women who are HPV-positive will all be treated, and VIA is used to determine eligibility for treatment with cryotherapy or LEEP.

b. In the 'HPV test followed by VIA' strategy, women who are HPV-negative are not treated. Women who are HPV-positive all undergo VIA, which is used in this case as a second screening test to determine treatment. Women who are HPV-positive and VIA-positive will all be treated, while women who are HPV-positive and VIA-negative will not be treated.

Screening intervals and follow-up

Ideal screening intervals are provided below and for all screen-and-treat strategies in Annexes 3 and 4.

In women who test negative on VIA or cytology (Pap smear), the screening interval for repeat screening should be every three to five years. In women who test negative on an HPV test, rescreening should be done after a minimum interval of five years. Women who have received treatment should receive post-treatment follow-up screening at one year to ensure effectiveness of treatment. Refer to Annex 3 for flowcharts for all strategies for women who are of negative or unknown HIV status.

In women who are of HIV-positive status or of unknown HIV status in areas with high endemic HIV infection, if the screening test is negative, the screening interval for repeat screening should be within three years. Women who have received treatment should receive post-treatment follow-up screening at one year to ensure effectiveness of treatment. Refer to Annex 4 for flowcharts for all strategies for women who are of HIV-positive status or of unknown HIV status in areas with high endemic HIV infection.

Screen-and-treat recommendations

Recommendation 1. The expert panel recommends against the use of CKC as treatment in a screen-and-treat strategy (strong recommendation, ⊕⊖⊖⊖ evidence)

Remarks: The screen-and-treat strategies considered by the panel with CKC as treatment included an HPV test, VIA, or an HPV test followed by VIA as screening. Although the benefits were similar for CKC compared with cryotherapy or LEEP for all screen-and-treat strategies, the harms were greater with CKC. This recommendation applies to women regardless of HIV status. See Supplemental material, Sections A and B.

Summary of the evidence: Low-quality evidence from pooled observational studies showed that the recurrence of CIN after treatment with CKC may be 3% less than the recurrence after cryotherapy or LEEP. However, this difference did not lead to important differences in cervical cancer incidence or related mortality (risk difference of 0.08%). In contrast, the incidence of major bleeding requiring hospitalization or blood transfusions may be greater (1/1000 treated with CKC versus 1/10 000 with cryotherapy or LEEP for most screen-and-treat strategies) and the risk of premature delivery after treatment with CKC may be greater than with cryotherapy or LEEP (Risk Ratio 3.41 versus 2.00). The increased risks of these complications apply to all treated women, regardless of whether they were correctly or incorrectly classified as having CIN2+ (i.e. including women with false-positive results who are treated unnecessarily). These differences were similar to the benefits and harms found when modelled for women of HIV-positive status.

Recommendation 2. Where resources permit, the expert panel suggests a strategy of screen with an HPV test and treat with cryotherapy (or LEEP when not eligible for cryotherapy) over a strategy of screen with VIA and treat with cryotherapy (or LEEP when not eligible) (conditional recommendation, ⊕⊖⊖⊖ evidence)

In resource-constrained settings, where screening with an HPV test is not feasible, the expert panel suggests a strategy of screen with VIA and treat with cryotherapy (or LEEP when not eligible) over a strategy of screen with an HPV test and treat with cryotherapy (or LEEP when not eligible) (conditional recommendation, ⊕⊖⊖⊖ evidence)

Remarks: The benefits of screen-and-treat with an HPV test or VIA, compared to no screening, outweighed the harms, but the reductions in cancer and related mortality were greater with an HPV test when compared to VIA. The availability of HPV testing is resource-dependent and, therefore, the expert panel suggests that an HPV test over VIA be provided where it is available, affordable, implementable, and sustainable over time. This recommendation applies to women regardless of HIV status. See Supplemental material, Sections A and B.

Summary of the evidence: Low-quality to very-low-quality evidence showed that there may be fewer CIN2+ recurrences with the screen-and-treat strategy using an HPV test (3/1000 fewer), as well as fewer cervical cancers (1/10 000 fewer) and fewer deaths (6/100 000 fewer) than with a strategy using VIA for screening. These differences result from fewer missed cases of CIN2+ with the HPV test strategy compared with the VIA strategy (i.e. fewer false negatives). The difference in overtreatment may be relatively small (157 000 cases with an HPV test versus 127 000 cases with VIA out of 1 000 000 women). The number of cancers found at first-time screening may be slightly greater with VIA (7/10 000 more). There may be little to no difference in complications, such as major bleeding or infections (e.g. 1/100 000 fewer with the VIA strategy). These results are similar to the benefits and harms found when modelled for women of HIV-positive status.

Recommendation 3. The expert panel suggests a strategy of screen with an HPV test and treat with cryotherapy (or LEEP when not eligible for cryotherapy) over a strategy of screen with cytology followed by colposcopy (with or without biopsy) and treat with cryotherapy (or LEEP when not eligible) (conditional recommendation, ⊕⊖⊖⊖ evidence)

Remarks: The reductions in cancer and related mortality were slightly greater with an HPV test only compared to cytology followed by colposcopy. Although there may be overtreatment of populations with high HPV prevalence and consequently more harms, as well as fewer cancers seen at first-time screening with an HPV test, there are greater resources required in cytology programmes due to quality control, training, and waiting time. The addition of colposcopy also requires a second visit. However, in countries where an appropriate/high-quality screening strategy with cytology (referring women with ASCUS or greater results) followed by colposcopy already exists, either an HPV test or cytology followed by colposcopy could be used. See Supplemental material, Sections A and B.

Summary of the evidence: As there were few to no studies evaluating the diagnostic accuracy of cytology followed by colposcopy compared to an HPV test, the effects of the sequence of tests were calculated by combining diagnostic data from cytology and colposcopy, resulting in lower-quality evidence. For the strategy of cytology followed by colposcopy (with or without biopsy), we analysed data for two scenarios: (1) Women who screened positive on cytology underwent colposcopy only (i.e. treatment was based on colposcopic impression); and (2) Women who screened positive on cytology underwent colposcopy, and then women with positive colposcopy results were biopsied (i.e. treatment was based on the biopsy result). Evidence showed that there may be fewer CIN2+ recurrences with the HPV test strategy (3/1000 fewer), as well as fewer cervical cancers (1/10 000 fewer) and fewer deaths (6/100 000 fewer) than with cytology followed by colposcopy. These differences result from fewer missed cases of CIN2+ with the HPV test strategy (i.e. fewer false negatives). Overtreatment, however, may be slightly greater with an HPV test when compared with cytology followed by colposcopy without biopsy (7/100 more women) or with biopsy when indicated (10/100 more women). This may result in slightly more complications with the HPV test strategy. The number of cancers detected at first-time screening may be slightly greater with the cytology followed by colposcopy strategy (1/1000 more).

Recommendation 4. The expert panel recommends a strategy of screen with VIA and treat with cryotherapy (or LEEP when not eligible for cryotherapy) over a strategy of screen with cytology followed by colposcopy (with or without biopsy) and treat with cryotherapy (or LEEP when not eligible) (strong recommendation, ⊕⊖⊖⊖ evidence)

Remarks: The benefits and harms of the two screen-and-treat strategies are similar, but there are fewer harms with cytology followed by colposcopy with biopsy when indicated. Despite overtreatment with VIA and fewer cancers detected at first-time screening, more resources are required for cytology programmes with colposcopy (with or without biopsy) due to quality control, training, and waiting time, as well as a second visit. The recommendation for VIA over cytology followed by colposcopy can be applied in countries that are currently considering either strategy, or countries that currently have both strategies available. This recommendation applies to women regardless of HIV status. See Supplemental material, Sections A and B.

Summary of the evidence: As there were few to no studies evaluating the diagnostic accuracy of cytology followed by colposcopy compared to VIA, the effects of the sequence of tests were calculated by combining diagnostic data from cytology and colposcopy, resulting in lower-quality evidence. For the strategy of cytology followed by colposcopy (with or without biopsy), we analysed data for two scenarios: (1) Women who screened positive on cytology underwent colposcopy only (i.e. treatment was based on colposcopic impression); and (2) Women who screened positive on cytology underwent colposcopy, and then women with positive colposcopy results were biopsied (i.e. treatment was based on the biopsy result). Evidence showed that there may be little or no difference in CIN2+ recurrence, cervical cancers, and related mortality between the strategies. Overtreatment, however, may be slightly greater with VIA compared to cytology followed by colposcopy without biopsy (11/100 more women) or with biopsy when indicated (18/100 more women). This may result in slightly greater harm with the VIA strategy. The number of cancers detected at first-time screening may be slightly greater with the cytology followed by colposcopy strategy (2/1000 more) compared with the VIA strategy.

Recommendation 5. The expert panel suggests a strategy of screen with an HPV test and treat with cryotherapy (or LEEP when not eligible for cryotherapy) over a strategy of screen with an HPV test followed by colposcopy (with or without biopsy) and treat with cryotherapy (or LEEP when not eligible) (conditional recommendation, ⊕⊖⊖⊖ evidence)

Remarks: The reductions in cancer and related mortality with either strategy outweigh the harms and costs of no screening, and were similar between the two strategies. Although overtreatment and, consequently, harms are reduced with the addition of colposcopy (with or without biopsy), there are more resource implications with colposcopy due to increased training of providers, quality control, waiting time, and the potential for more women to be lost to follow-up. The addition of colposcopy to an HPV test would also require a second visit. In countries without an existing screening strategy, an HPV test followed by colposcopy is not recommended. This recommendation applies to women regardless of HIV status. See Supplemental material, Sections A and B.

Summary of the evidence: As there were few to no studies evaluating the diagnostic accuracy of an HPV test followed by colposcopy, the effects of the sequence of tests were calculated by combining diagnostic data from the individual tests, resulting in lower-quality evidence. For the strategy of an HPV test followed by colposcopy (with or without biopsy), we analysed data for two scenarios: (1) Women who screened positive on HPV testing underwent colposcopy only (i.e. treatment was based on colposcopic impression); and (2) Women who screened positive on HPV testing underwent colposcopy, and then women with positive colposcopy results were biopsied (i.e. treatment was based on the biopsy result). Evidence showed that there may be little to no difference in CIN2+ recurrence, cervical cancers, and related mortality between the strategies. Overtreatment, however, may be slightly greater with an HPV test only compared with an HPV test followed by colposcopy without biopsy (5/100 more women) or with biopsy when indicated (12/100 more women). This may result in slightly greater harm with an HPV-test-only strategy. The number of cancers detected at first-time screening may be slightly greater with an HPV test followed by colposcopy strategy (1/1000 more) than with an HPV test only.

Recommendation 6. The expert panel suggests either a strategy of screen with an HPV test followed by VIA and treat with cryotherapy (or LEEP when not eligible for cryotherapy) or a strategy of screen with an HPV test and treat with cryotherapy (or LEEP when not eligible) (conditional recommendation, ⊕⊖⊖⊖ evidence)

Remarks: The reductions in cancer and related mortality were greater with an HPV test used as a single screening test than with an HPV test followed by VIA, and this reduction was even greater in women of HIV-positive status. However, there may be overtreatment, and thus potentially greater harms with screen-and-treat when using an HPV test as a single test. There is also some uncertainty about the effects of an HPV test followed by VIA and how VIA performs after a positive HPV test because there was no direct evidence about this strategy. There is also the potential for additional resources that are required to refer women for VIA testing after a positive HPV test, the need for a second visit to perform VIA, and increased training to perform both tests. For these reasons, the recommendation is for either an HPV test followed by VIA or an HPV test only, and it is conditional. It is to be noted that benefits are more pronounced compared to harm in women of HIV-positive status when using an HPV test only. See Supplemental material, Sections A and B.

Summary of the evidence: As there were no studies evaluating the diagnostic accuracy of an HPV test followed by VIA, the effects were calculated by combining diagnostic data from an HPV test only with data for VIA only, resulting in lower-quality evidence. This evidence showed that there may be slightly greater CIN2+ recurrences with an HPV test followed by VIA (4/1000 more), as well as more cervical cancers (1/10 000 more) and more deaths (7/100 000 more) than with an HPV test only. The difference was due to a slightly higher rate of missed cases of CIN 2+ with an HPV test followed by VIA than with an HPV test only (6/1000 more). The number of cancers detected at first-time screening may be slightly greater with an HPV test followed by VIA (7/10 000 more), and there may be fewer women treated unnecessarily (1/10 fewer) due to the lower false-positive rate with an HPV test followed by VIA. If fewer women are treated unnecessarily, this may result in lower resource use and fewer complications with an HPV test followed by VIA.

However, these results were more pronounced when modelled for women of HIV-positive status. There may be greater differences in benefits and harms. The evidence for women of HIV-positive status showed that there is likely to be an even greater rate of CIN2+ recurrences with an HPV test followed by VIA (22/1000 more), as well as more cervical cancers (17/10 000 more) and more deaths (12/100 000 more) than with HPV only. However, there may be fewer women treated unnecessarily (1/10 fewer) when using the screening strategy of an HPV test followed by VIA, resulting in fewer resources for unnecessary treatment and fewer complications.

Recommendation 7. The expert panel suggests a strategy of screen with an HPV test followed by VIA and treat with cryotherapy (or LEEP when not eligible for cryotherapy) over a strategy of screen with VIA and treat with cryotherapy (or LEEP when not eligible) (conditional recommendation, ⊕⊖⊖⊖ evidence)

Remarks: The reductions in cancer and related mortality with an HPV test followed by VIA or with VIA alone outweighed the harms. However, the harms may be greater when using VIA only, which is likely due to overtreatment. Although a slightly larger number of cancers may be detected on initial screen with VIA only. This recommendation is conditional due to the uncertain costs of providing the sequence of two tests (HPV test followed by VIA) over the single VIA test. In countries where an HPV test is not available, we suggest screening with VIA only. This recommendation applies to women regardless of HIV status. See Supplemental material, Sections A and B.

Summary of the evidence: As there were no studies evaluating the diagnostic accuracy of an HPV test followed by VIA, the effects were calculated by combining diagnostic data from an HPV test only with data for VIA only, resulting in lower-quality evidence. This evidence showed little to no difference in CIN2+ recurrence, cervical cancer, and related mortality between a screen-and-treat strategy using an HPV test followed by VIA and a strategy using VIA only. This was likely due to the relatively small differences in the number of missed cases of CIN2+ between the two strategies. Although the number of cancers detected at first-time screening may be slightly greater with VIA only (7/10 000 more), there may be more women treated unnecessarily (1/10 more) due to higher false-positive rates with VIA only (incurring higher resource use for overtreatment). Overtreatment may also result in greater complications with VIA only. These results are similar to the benefits and harms found when modelled for women of HIV-positive status.

Recommendation 8. The expert panel suggests a strategy of screen with an HPV test followed by VIA and treat with cryotherapy (or LEEP when not eligible for cryotherapy) over a strategy of screen with cytology followed by colposcopy (with or without biopsy) and treat with cryotherapy (or LEEP when not eligible) (conditional recommendation, ⊕⊖⊖⊖ evidence)

Remarks: The benefits of the two screen-and-treat strategies are similar. However, there may be higher resources required in cytology programmes due to quality control, training, and waiting time. The addition of colposcopy requires a second visit. This recommendation applies to women regardless of HIV status. See Supplemental material, Sections A and B.

Summary of the evidence: As there were few to no studies evaluating the diagnostic accuracy of cytology followed by colposcopy compared to an HPV test followed by VIA, the effects of the sequence of tests were calculated by combining diagnostic data, resulting in lower-quality evidence. For the strategy of cytology followed by colposcopy (with or without biopsy), we analysed data for two scenarios: (1) Women who screened positive on cytology underwent colposcopy only (i.e. treatment was based on colposcopic impression); and (2) Women who screened positive on cytology underwent colposcopy, and then women with positive colposcopy results were biopsied (i.e. treatment was based on the biopsy result). Evidence showed that there may be little to no difference in CIN2+ recurrence, cervical cancers, and related mortality between the strategies. There may also be little to no difference in overtreatment between the strategies. The number of cancers detected at first-time screening may be slightly greater with the cytology followed by colposcopy strategy (2/1000 more).

Recommendation 9. The expert panel suggests a strategy of screen with an HPV test followed by VIA and treat with cryotherapy (or LEEP when not eligible for cryotherapy) over a strategy of screen with an HPV test followed by colposcopy (with or without biopsy) and treat with cryotherapy (or LEEP when not eligible) (conditional recommendation, ⊕⊖⊖⊖ evidence)

Remarks: The reductions in cancer and related mortality of screen-and-treat with an HPV test followed by colposcopy (with or without biopsy) may be slightly greater compared to an HPV test followed by VIA. The panel agreed that the benefits of either strategy outweigh the harms and costs; however, the difference in costs between the strategies is uncertain. There may be more resource implications with colposcopy due to increased training of providers, quality control, waiting time, and the potential for more women to be lost to follow-up. It is also unclear whether women would perceive a difference between VIA and colposcopy; however, a biopsy during colposcopy may be less acceptable than VIA. This recommendation applies to women regardless of HIV status. See Supplemental material, Sections A and B.

Summary of the evidence: As there were few to no studies evaluating the diagnostic accuracy of both screening strategies, the effects of the strategies were calculated by combining diagnostic data from the individual tests, resulting in lower-quality evidence. For the strategy of an HPV test followed by colposcopy (with or without biopsy), we analysed data for two scenarios: (1) Women who screened positive on HPV testing underwent colposcopy only (i.e. treatment was based on colposcopic impression); and (2) Women who screened positive on HPV testing underwent colposcopy, and then women with positive colposcopy results were biopsied (i.e. treatment was based on the biopsy result). Evidence showed that there may be fewer CIN2+ recurrences with the HPV test followed by colposcopy without biopsy (3/1000 fewer) and with biopsy (4/1000 fewer), as well as fewer cervical cancers (1/10 000 fewer with or without biopsy) and fewer deaths (6/100 000 fewer, with or without biopsy) than with an HPV test followed by VIA. These differences result from fewer missed cases of CIN2+ with the HPV test followed by colposcopy strategy when compared to an HPV test followed by VIA strategy (i.e. fewer false negatives). Overtreatment, however, may be greater with an HPV test followed by colposcopy without biopsy than with an HPV test followed by VIA (7/100 more women). There may be little to no difference between the strategies in the number of cancers detected at first-time screening.

4. Research gaps and further considerations

The best evidence to assess the effects of a screen-and-treat strategy is from randomized controlled trials in which women are randomly allocated to receive one or another screen-and-treat strategy and then all screened women are followed and patient-important health outcomes – such as CIN recurrence, cervical cancer and complications of treatment – are measured. We identified few randomized controlled trials that evaluated screen-and-treat strategies and patient-important outcomes. In particular, there were very few studies that assessed the strategies that the GDG ranked as clinically relevant (e.g. HPV test followed by VIA). In fact, few studies were found, randomized controlled trials or otherwise, that assessed a sequence of tests, such as an HPV test followed by VIA. There were also few studies that assessed the accuracy of diagnostic tests or reported on patient outcomes in women who are HIV-positive or at high risk of being HIV-positive.

There is some concern about the use of cytology programmes in areas where health systems are not robust, resources are limited, or quality assurance is not maintained. Cytology programmes have been and remain difficult to establish in low- and middle-income settings. Quality assurance to ensure accurate and reproducible results in cytology programmes requires greater human and financial resources than other screening strategies, and, as cytology results are not available quickly, there is a greater chance of women being lost to follow-up, which reduces the benefits of cytology-based programmes. Cytology followed by colposcopy (with or without biopsy) was not shown in this review of the literature to lead to better outcomes as compared with other screening strategies for cervical cancer prevention. Using another screening test, such as an HPV test, prior to cytology was also not investigated in this evidence review, nor modelled for these recommendations.

Although the potential value of a screen-and-treat algorithm focusing on HPV testing followed by cytology is of interest to some workers in this area, the expert panel did not rank an exploration of this algorithm highly enough for it to be among the PICO questions (population, intervention, comparison, outcome) addressed as part of the process of preparing these guidelines. This was largely due to the fact that, for the audience likely to benefit most from these guidelines, the expert panel felt that questions concerning cytology were not as germane to programme guidance as questions relating to HPV and VIA testing coupled with cryotherapy. Another reason was that there was consensus among the expert panel that adding a cytology component could place significant constraints on the intent to have expeditious links between testing and treatment. Therefore an evidence base on the question of an HPV test followed by cytology was not developed and no recommendations on this algorithm are offered at present. Once studies become available that provide rigorous comparisons between, for example, an HPV test/cytology and an HPV test/VIA (or vice versa), then these could be the focus of a subsequent GRADE analysis, which could then generate evidence-based recommendations.

These recommendations make a distinction between the use of VIA as a method to determine eligibility for treatment with cryotherapy or LEEP and the use of VIA to determine whether to treat or not (see explanation in Chapter 3, under the subheading *Considerations for treatments*). When VIA is used following a positive test for HPV, women are treated only if they are also VIA-positive. However, there are few studies that evaluated the overall diagnostic test accuracy of this sequence of screening tests or measured patient-important outcomes after providing this sequence of tests. There are also no studies that compare outcomes when using VIA to determine eligibility for cryotherapy.

The GDG also made a distinction between the use of 'colposcopic impression' versus 'colposcopic impression and biopsy when indicated'. In the former, a woman who was positive on a first screening test would be treated only if the visualization by colposcopy was positive for a lesion. However, in the latter, a positive colposcopy would be followed by a biopsy and only women with a positive biopsy would be treated (essentially not a screen-and-treat strategy). Again, this sequence of tests was not evaluated or compared in randomized controlled trials, nor was any evidence available from observational diagnostic test accuracy studies. Therefore modelling was used to determine if eliminating the biopsy step from the strategy would still result in similar net benefits, while reducing the use of resources.

Because few randomized controlled trials evaluated screen-and-treat strategies, the MG used a model and therefore needed data about the baseline risks and the natural history of the disease. Data for the natural progression and regression of CIN2+ across women of many age groups and for women of HIV-positive status were all unclear. While there are ethical issues to consider, it should be possible to conduct studies that follow women over longer periods of time. Due to the lack of such data, it was challenging to determine the age at which screening should be started and ended, and how often rescreening should occur. There were many unanswered questions about women aged 20–35 years, and women over the age of 50, and about the optimal intervals for follow-up after treatment. Yet the recommendations included in this guideline are based on modelling scenarios that illustrate what age groups, what screening frequency, and what follow-up period has the greatest impact on cervical cancer mortality.

Lastly, the GDG identified and prioritized outcomes for screen-and-treat strategies that were important to the decision-making process. For many of these outcomes, there was low-quality to very-low-quality evidence, and only indirect evidence. The GDG identified, in particular, fertility and reproductive outcomes as a concern for many women. Also of concern was HIV transmission, but there is little research measuring this outcome. Other benefits of screening were also identified by the GDG, such as the detection of sexually transmitted infections or the detection of cervical cancer, which may be dependent on the screening test used (e.g. HPV test versus VIA). However, these benefits are not currently or consistently measured in studies.

5. Use of the guideline

Guideline dissemination

These guidelines will be available online at the WHO Library database and there will be a link on WHO's Sexual and Reproductive Health web page and in the *WHO Reproductive Health Library* (RHL), an electronic review journal.[7] The publication will also be announced in the UNDP/UNFPA/UNICEF/WHO/World Bank Special Programme of Research, Development and Research Training in Human Reproduction (HRP) *WHO Reproductive Health Update*,[8] which reaches more than 2000 subscribers and numerous organizations with whom we are working. Many of these organizations will also copy the announcement in their newsletters.

The guidelines will be distributed in print to subscribers to WHO publications, to the WHO mailing list for mandatory free distribution (national chief health executives, ministers of health or director-generals of health, depository libraries for WHO publications, WHO representatives/liaison officers, WHO/HQ library, WHO regional offices, and off-site office libraries), additional non-mandatory free recipients (competent national authorities for sexual and reproductive health, cancer control programmes, national research centres in reproductive health, and WHO collaborating centres), WHO staff at headquarters, regional and country offices and elsewhere, concerned NGOs, medical societies concerned with cancer control and/or sexual and reproductive health, scientific journals (including general medical journals and journals specialized on sexual and reproductive health or cancer), international organizations, and donors, potential donors, potential publishers of translated versions, as well as all those who contributed to the documents.

Conference invitations to discuss and present the guidelines will be accepted.

Regional conferences are already planned in the Americas and Africa to present the new recommendations to a number of stakeholders involved in national programme planning in 2013. The other regions will be covered in 2014.

If requested by regional offices, countries will be supported to adapt the guideline to their country-specific needs and to integrate the material with existing national guidelines. Adaptation will be done by organizing regional, sub-regional and country-level workshops for discussion of each recommendation, in order to adapt them to the national epidemiologic, cultural, and socioeconomic context.

Initially, the guidelines will be available in English only and translations will be developed subject to the availability of funding. Translation into non-UN languages and publication in these languages by third parties will be encouraged.

Guideline evaluation

The number of downloads from the WHO web sites (headquarters and regional) will be used as an indicator of interest in these guidelines.

We are working with the WHO regional offices to monitor requests from countries for technical assistance to use these guidelines. For this purpose, national stakeholder meetings will be organized in-country, and feedback on the clarity, feasibility, and usefulness of the recommendations will be recorded.

We will also monitor, with the regional offices, how many countries change their recommendations based on the publication of these new recommendations for screen-and-treat strategies.

---

[7] The WHO Library database is available at http://www.who.int/library/databases/en/; WHO's Sexual and Reproductive Health web page is available at http://www.who.int/reproductivehealth/topics/cancers/en/index.html; WHO's RHL is available at: http://apps.who.int/rhl/en/.

[8] A subscription to HRP's *WHO Reproductive Health Update* can be requested at http://www.who.int/reproductivehealth/RHUpdate/en/index.html.

Guideline update

The GDG will continue to work with WHO in an ad hoc manner, so that the research gaps identified during the process can be addressed. In addition, evidence published on new screening and treatment methods will be monitored so that updates to these recommendations can be considered promptly. We anticipate that around five years after the publication of these recommendations sufficient new evidence will be available to update the present recommendations and potentially add new ones.

References

1. Arbyn M et al. Evidence regarding human papillomavirus testing in secondary prevention of cervical cancer. *Vaccine*, 2012, 30 Suppl 5: F88–99.

2. De Vuyst H et al. Prevalence and determinants of human papillomavirus infection and cervical lesions in HIV-positive women in Kenya. *British Journal of Cancer*, 2012, 107(9):1624–1630.

3. Denny L et al. Human papillomavirus infection and cervical disease in human immunodeficiency virus-1-infected women. *Obstetrics & Gynecology*, 2008, 111(6):1380–1387.

4. Joshi S et al. Screening of cervical neoplasia in HIV-infected women in India. *AIDS*, 2013, 27(4):607–615.

5. Zhang HY et al. HPV prevalence and cervical intraepithelial neoplasia among HIV-infected women in Yunnan Province, China: a pilot study. *Asian Pacific Journal of Cancer Prevention*, 2012, 13(1):91–96.

6. Santesso N et al.; World Health Organization Steering Committee for Recommendations on Use of Cryotherapy for Cervical Cancer Prevention. World Health Organization Guidelines: use of cryotherapy for cervical intraepithelial neoplasia. *International Journal of Gynecology & Obstetrics,* 2012, 118(2):97–102.

7. *WHO guidelines: use of cryotherapy for cervical intraepithelial neoplasia*. Geneva, World Health Organization, Department of Reproductive Health and Research, 2011 (http://www.who.int/reproductivehealth/publications/cancers/9789241502856/en/, accessed 24 October 2013).

8. *WHO guidelines for treatment of cervical intraepithelial neoplasia 2–3 and glandular adenocarcinoma in situ: Cryotherapy, large loop excision of the transformation zone (LEEP/LLETZ), and cold knife conization*. Geneva, World Health Organization (in process).

9. Sellors JW, Sankaranarayanan R. *Colposcopy and treatment of cervical intraepithelial neoplasia: a beginner's manual*. France, International Agency for Research on Cancer, World Health Organization, 2003 (http://screening.iarc.fr/doc/Colposcopymanual.pdf, accessed 24 October 2013).

10. *Comprehensive cervical cancer control: a guide to essential practice* (C4-GEP). Geneva, World Health Organization, Department of Reproductive Health and Research and Department of Chronic Diseases and Health Promotion, 2006 (http://www.who.int/reproductivehealth/publications/cancers/9241547006/en/, accessed 20 August 2013).

11. *WHO handbook for guideline development*. Geneva, World Health Organization, 2010 (http://www.who.int/hiv/topics/mtct/grc_handbook_mar2010_1.pdf, accessed 6 August 2013).

12. *WHO handbook for guideline development*. Geneva, World Health Organization, 2012 (http://apps.who.int/iris/bitstream/10665/75146/1/9789241548441_eng.pdf, accessed 6 August 2013).

13. Higgins JPT, Green S, eds. *Cochrane handbook for systematic reviews of interventions* Version 5.1.0. The Cochrane Collaboration, updated March 2011 (www.cochrane-handbook.org, accessed 6 August 2013).

14. Guyatt GH et al.; GRADE Working Group. GRADE: an emerging consensus on rating quality of evidence and strength of recommendations. *BMJ*, 2008, 336:924–926.

15. Schünemann HJ et al.; GRADE Working Group. Grading quality of evidence and strength of recommendations for diagnostic tests and strategies. *BMJ*, 2008, 336:1106–1110.

16. Bradley J et al. Women's perspectives on cervical screening and treatment in developing countries: experiences with new technologies and service delivery strategies. *Women and Health*, 2006, 43(3):103–121.

17. Melnikow J et al. Management of the low-grade abnormal Pap smear: what are women's preferences? *Journal of Family Practice*, 2002, 51(10):849–855.

18. Frederiksen ME, Lynge E, Rebolj M. What women want. Women's preferences for the management of low-grade abnormal cervical screening tests: a systematic review. *BJOG: An International Journal of Obstetrics and Gynaecology*, 2012, 119(1):7–19.

19. Chirenje ZM et al. A randomised clinical trial of loop electrosurgical excision procedure (LEEP) versus cryotherapy in the treatment of cervical intraepithelial neoplasia. *Journal of Obstetrics and Gynaecology*, 2001, 21(6):617–621.

20. *WHO cervical cancer prevention and control costing tool (C4P)*. Geneva, World Health Organization, 2012 (http://www.who.int/nuvi/hpv/cervical_cancer_costing_tool/en/index.html, accessed 24 October 2013).

Annex 1. Declarations of interest

Out of the 54 experts who participated in this work, 15 declared an interest related to cervical cancer. Although not all of these interests are specifically related to cervical cancer screening and treatment, they are nonetheless all disclosed and summarized below.

Marc Arbyn was invited by the European Research Organisation on Genital Infection and Neoplasia (EUROGIN) to speak at its 2011 conference in Lisbon. EUROGIN covered his travel and lodging expenses. EUROGIN is an organization that promotes and develops, at the level of the European region, research, training, screening, prevention and information concerning genital infections, pre-cancers and cancers in women. EUROGIN conferences are financially supported by a range of pharmaceutical companies with an interest in cervical cancer.

Paul Blumenthal was the principal investigator of an operations research study conducted by the Department of Obstetrics and Gynecology at Stanford University School of Medicine to evaluate the feasibility and acceptability of introducing a new rapid HPV test (careHPV) manufactured by Qiagen for low- and middle-income settings. Qiagen lent the equipment and provided the tests for this research.

John-Paul Bogers is employed by the University of Antwerp and acts as a consultant for SonicHealthcare Benelux to perform clinical pathology work and validate new technologies in the field of treatment of cervical intraepithelial neoplasia (CIN). SonicHealthcare Benelux is a commercial laboratory that inter alia performs cervical cancer (cytology and HPV) screening. Bogers has also performed work for three other companies with an interest in cervical cancer screening: (1) an analytical validation of an HPV test for Innogenetics (contract value: €60 000); (2) an analytical validation of a Becton-Dickinson (BD) pathway machine (contract value: €10 000); and (3) a literature review in the field of treatment of CIN for Hologic (contract value: €5000).

August Burns is the Executive Director of Grounds for Health, a non-profit organization that aims to create sustainable and effective cervical cancer prevention and treatment programmes in coffee-growing communities, with the goal of decreasing the rate of cervical cancer. To support its projects, Grounds for Health received US$ 15 000 from the Union Internationale Contre le Cancer (UICC), a nongovernmental, non-profit organization that inter alia receives funding from companies with an interest in cancer.

Lynette Denny has spoken on HPV vaccination at various speakers' forums organized by the companies GlaxoSmithKline (GSK) and Merck. The honoraria for these activities amounted to approximately US$ 4000 per company per year and were paid to her employer, the University of Cape Town. The Department of Obstetrics and Gynaecology of the University of Cape Town, of which Denny is the head, has furthermore conducted two HPV vaccine trials for GSK and Merck. For these trials the University of Cape Town received US$ 1.6 million from GSK, but no funding from Merck as that funding was paid to the Department of Health, KwaZulu Natal. All work done on the project by Denny was done pro bono. Denny gave a talk on cost-effectiveness of HPV testing in Hong Kong, in 2012, and Qiagen paid for her registration, travel and accommodation. Denny is currently running a trial for Roche on the ability of the cobas® 4800 System to detect cancer – the cost is US$ 25 000. All the funds received by Denny either as a principal investigator or as a speaker are paid entirely to the University of Cape Town research accounts.

Silvia de Sanjosé has received occasional travel support from Sanofi, Merck and Qiagen to attend and present results of studies coordinated by her institution at national and international conferences. The amounts ranged from approximately US$ 1000 to US$ 3000 per trip, depending on the location of the conference. None of the funders had any role in the presentation of results. Some research studies in which de Sanjosé participates have been partially supported by GSK, Sanofi Pasteur MSD, Qiagen, Roche and Merck & Co., Inc., representing over US$ 100 000 a year for the last four years. None of the funders have had any role in the data collection, analysis or interpretation of the results.

Eduardo Franco has participated in advisory board meetings and forums relating to cervical cancer prevention strategies organized by Merck, Roche and Gen-Probe (either on HPV vaccines or HPV tests). He has received an average honorarium of US$ 4000 per company for these activities over the last four years.

Julia Gage has, as part of her work for the United States National Cancer Institute (NCI) of the National Institutes of Health (NIH), conducted an operations research project in Nigeria to evaluate the effectiveness of the careHPV screening test manufactured by Qiagen. Qiagen donated and shipped the reagents, equipment and supplies. NCI paid for all other aspects of the study.

Francisco Garcia was the principal investigator for drug trials of novel agents for the treatment of cervical cancer while he was employed at the University of Arizona. These trials were conducted by the University of Arizona under research contracts with Roche (US$ 150 000), Innovio (US$ 70 000), Photocure (US$ 120 000) and Roche/Ventana (US$ 100 000). Garcia did not receive any personal income for these trials.

José Jeronimo is an employee of PATH, an international non-profit organization involved in the development and delivery of high-impact, low-cost tools for global health. PATH has concluded collaborative research and development agreements for the development of a rapid HPV test with Qiagen (careHPV) and a rapid test for cervical cancer screening with Arbor Vita (identification of the E6 and E7 oncoproteins). PATH has received samples and equipment from both companies to conduct studies in different countries for the validation of these tests. In the PATH–Qiagen agreement, the commercialization of the test in China and India is considered a priority, with other countries to be included according to the conditions in each geographical area. These tests will be made available at low cost to the public sector in low-resource countries.

Enriquito Lu was the principal investigator of an HPV vaccination study conducted by his employer, the international, non-profit organization Jhpiego, under agreement with Merck. The purpose of the study was to evaluate the feasibility and acceptability of a strategy to deliver comprehensive cervical cancer prevention services in Thailand and the Philippines by integrating HPV vaccination for girls aged 9–13 into screening and treatment programmes for mothers. For this purpose, Jhpiego received from Merck US$ 850 000 and HPV vaccines for up to 4000 girls in each country project site. Lu did not receive any personal income for his work on this study.

Raul Murillo was a consultant for GSK to analyse the cost-effectiveness of the HPV vaccine. He received a total honorarium of US$ 5000 for this consultancy (which ended in 2010).

Swee Chong Queck has, over the past four years, participated in advisory board meetings and speakers' forums organized by GSK and Qiagen. These meetings and forums related to cervical cancer prevention strategies, HPV vaccine efficacy studies and clinical relevance of HPV vaccination for the prevention of cervical cancer and other HPV-related diseases. The total combined income received by Queck for these activities over the last four years was S$ 9000 (Singapore dollars).

Achim Schneider serves as an advisor to the company Karl Storz in the development of laparoscopic techniques and instruments for the treatment of cervical cancer and other benign or malignant diseases, for which he receives an annual honorarium of €40 000. Schneider has also participated in advisory board meetings and lectures relating to HPV vaccination, organized by GSK and Sanofi, respectively. For these latter activities he has received a total combined income of US$ 20 000 over the last four years.

Vivien Tsu is an employee of PATH, an international non-profit organization involved in the development and delivery of high-impact, low-cost tools for global health. As such, Tsu was involved in: (1) large-scale demonstration projects on the prevention, screening and treatment of cervical cancer in developing countries for which PATH received donated vaccine from GSK and Merck and careHPV tests from Qiagen; and (2) an alternative-dose-schedule study in Viet Nam, for which PATH received donated vaccine from Merck.

Annex 2. Decision-making flowchart for screen-and-treat strategies

This decision-making flowchart or algorithm provides a decision tree to use as a quick reference when choosing a screen-and-treat strategy at the programme level. Programme managers and decision-makers can start at the top and answer the questions accordingly to determine which screen-and-treat option is best in the context where it will be implemented. It highlights choices related to resources, which can include costs, staff and training. However, programme managers will also need to consider other factors, such as the number of women who are lost to follow-up with a strategy that involves more than one screening test. Refer to the screen-and-treat recommendations provided in Chapter 3 of the guideline for more specific guidance about which strategies are recommended, and for information on the specific factors to consider when deciding on a strategy. For details about the flow of each screen-and-treat strategy (e.g. HPV followed by VIA), consult the flowcharts in Annex 3 (for women of negative or unknown HIV status) and Annex 4 (for women of HIV-positive status or unknown HIV status in areas with high endemic HIV infection).

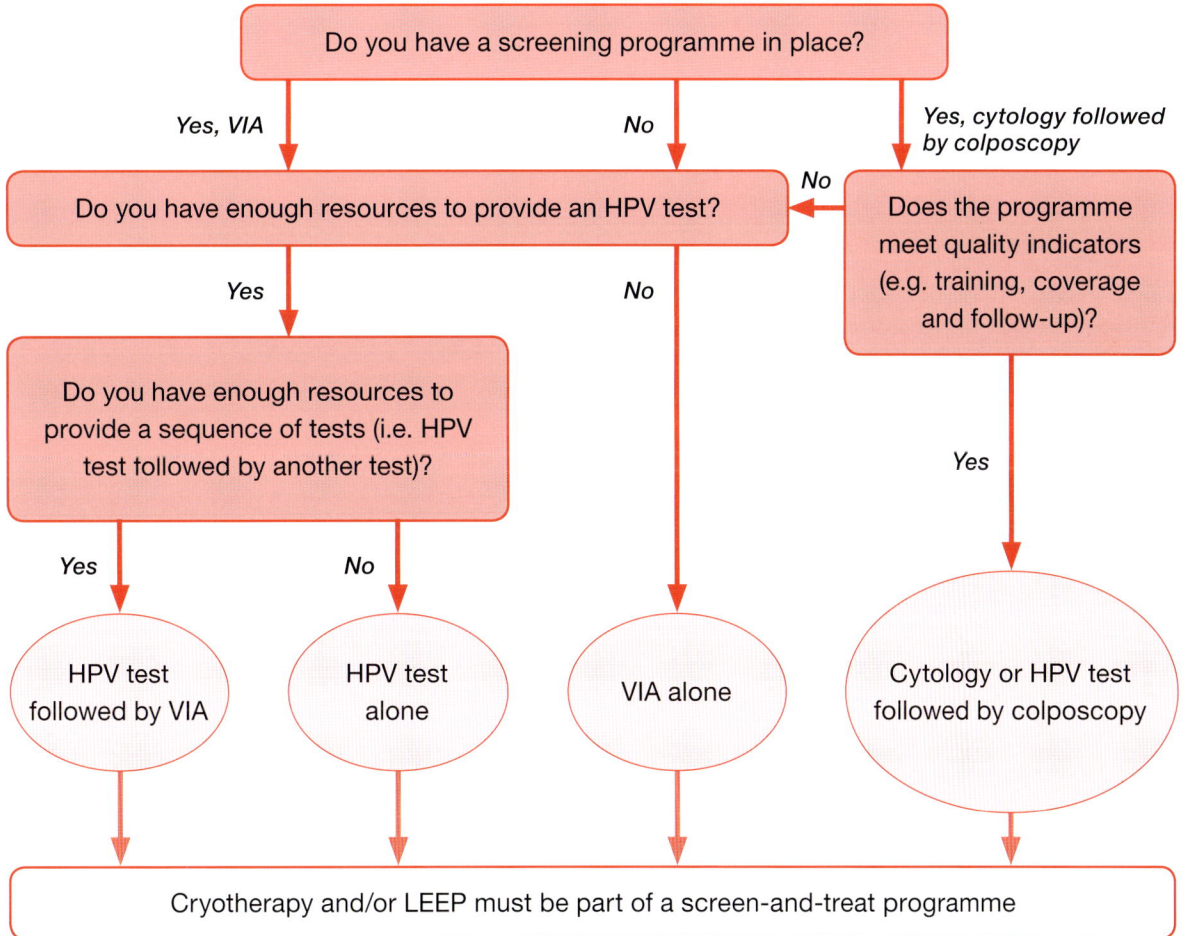

Note: each light-pink bubble refers to one strategy in Annex 3 (for women of negative or unknown HIV status) or Annex 4 (for women of HIV-positive status or unknown HIV status in areas with high endemic HIV infection)

Annex 3. Flowcharts for screen-and-treat strategies (negative or unknown HIV status)

The following flowcharts describe the steps for each of the screen-and-treat strategies that are available. The flowcharts *do not* indicate which strategy is preferred. Refer to the screen-and-treat recommendations provided in Chapter 3 of the guideline for guidance about which strategies are recommended, and to the decision-making flowchart in Annex 2. For detailed information about the specific factors the guideline panel considered when making the recommendations, refer to the evidence-to-recommendation tables for each recommendation (Supplemental material, Sections A and B).

Screen with an HPV test and treat with cryotherapy, or LEEP when not eligible for cryotherapy

When an HPV test is positive, treatment is provided. With this strategy, visual inspection with acetic acid (VIA) is used to determine **eligibility** for cryotherapy.

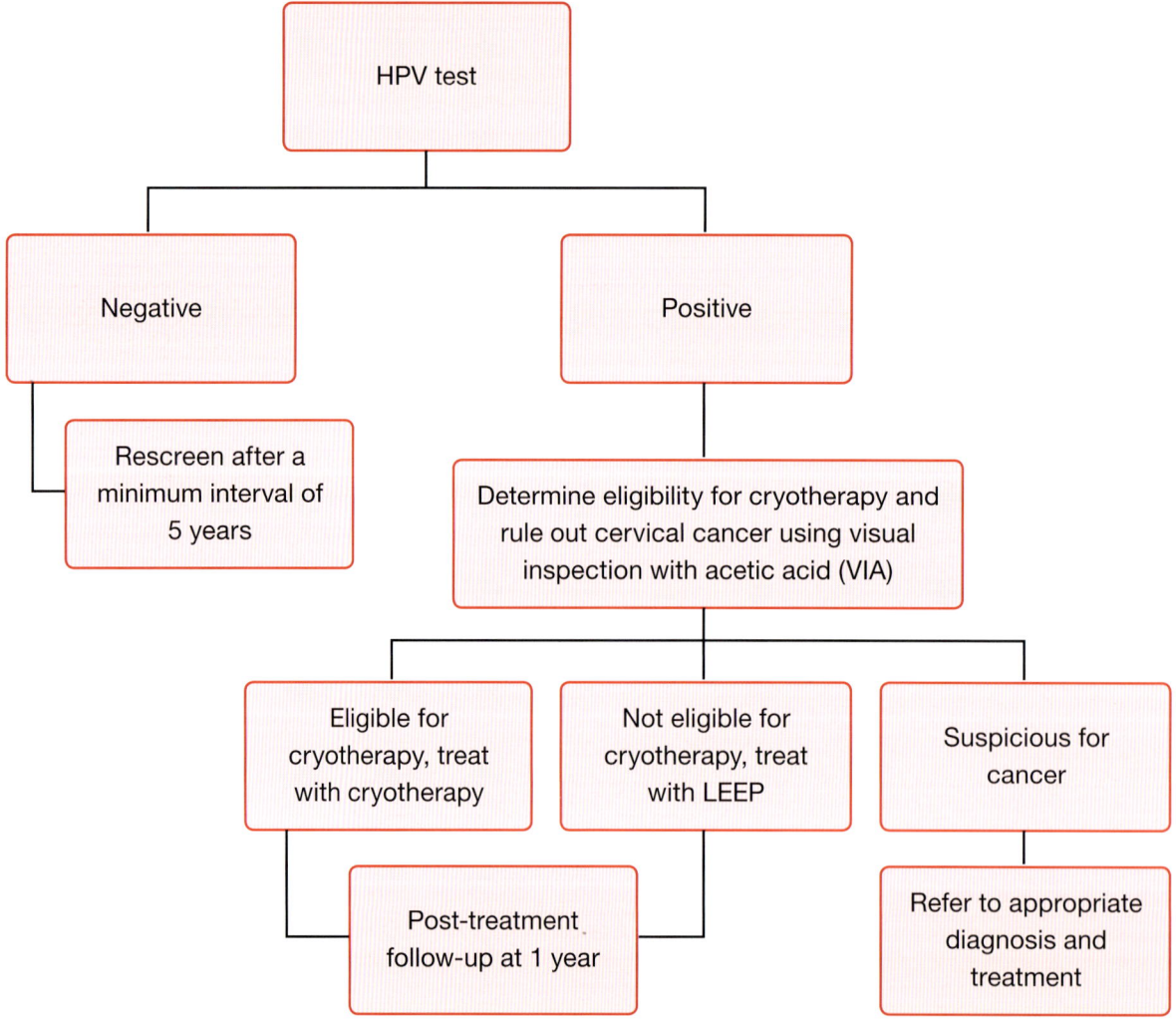

Note: Refer to the screen-and-treat recommendations provided in Chapter 3 of the guideline for guidance about which strategies are recommended, and for information on the specific factors to consider when deciding on a strategy.

Screen with an HPV test followed by VIA and treat with cryotherapy, or LEEP when not eligible for cryotherapy

When an HPV test is positive, then VIA is provided as a second screening test to determine whether or not treatment is offered. Treatment is only provided if BOTH the HPV test and VIA are positive.

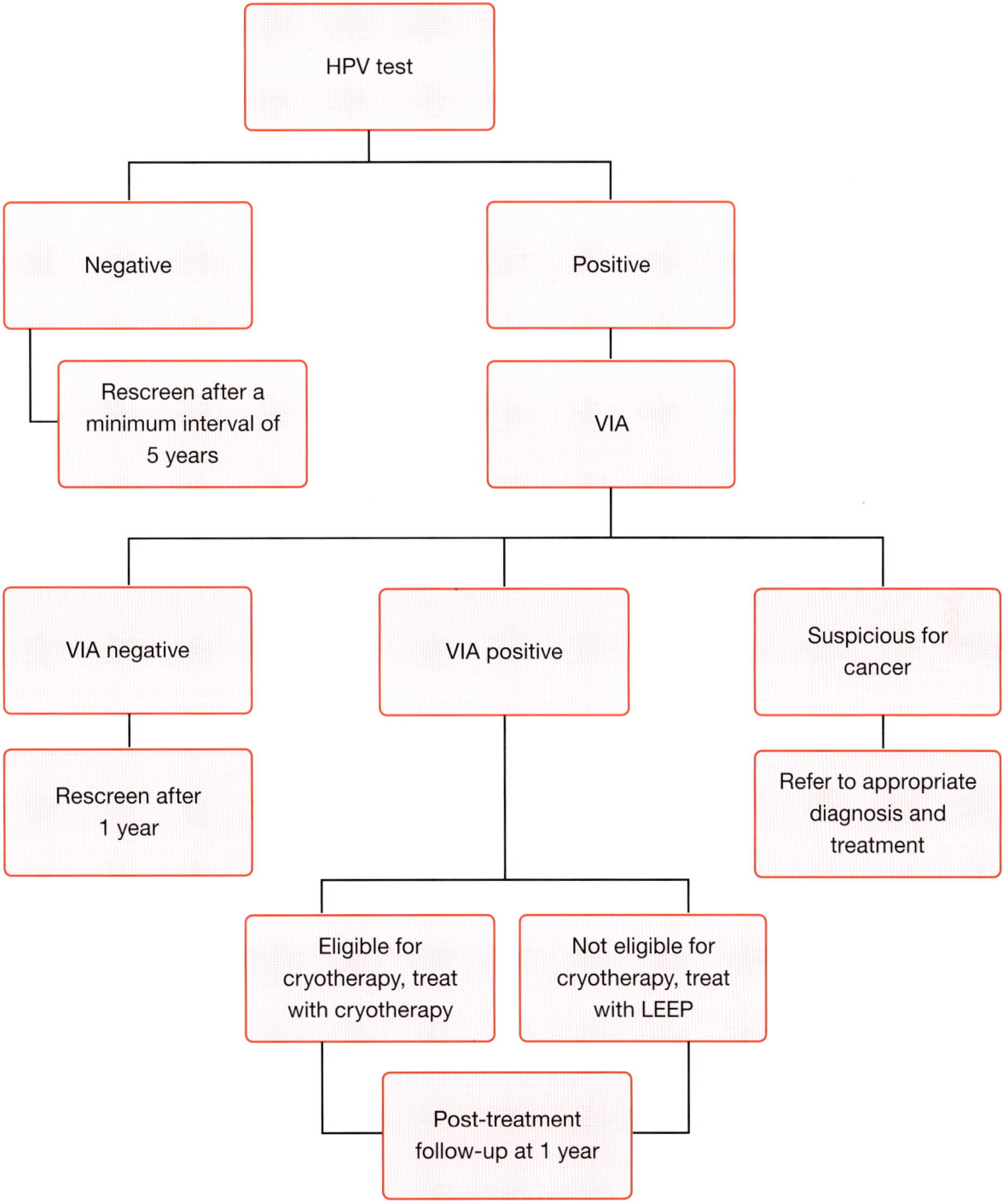

Note: Refer to the screen-and-treat recommendations provided in Chapter 3 of the guideline for guidance about which strategies are recommended, and for information on the specific factors to consider when deciding on a strategy.

Screen with VIA and treat with cryotherapy, or LEEP when not eligible for cryotherapy

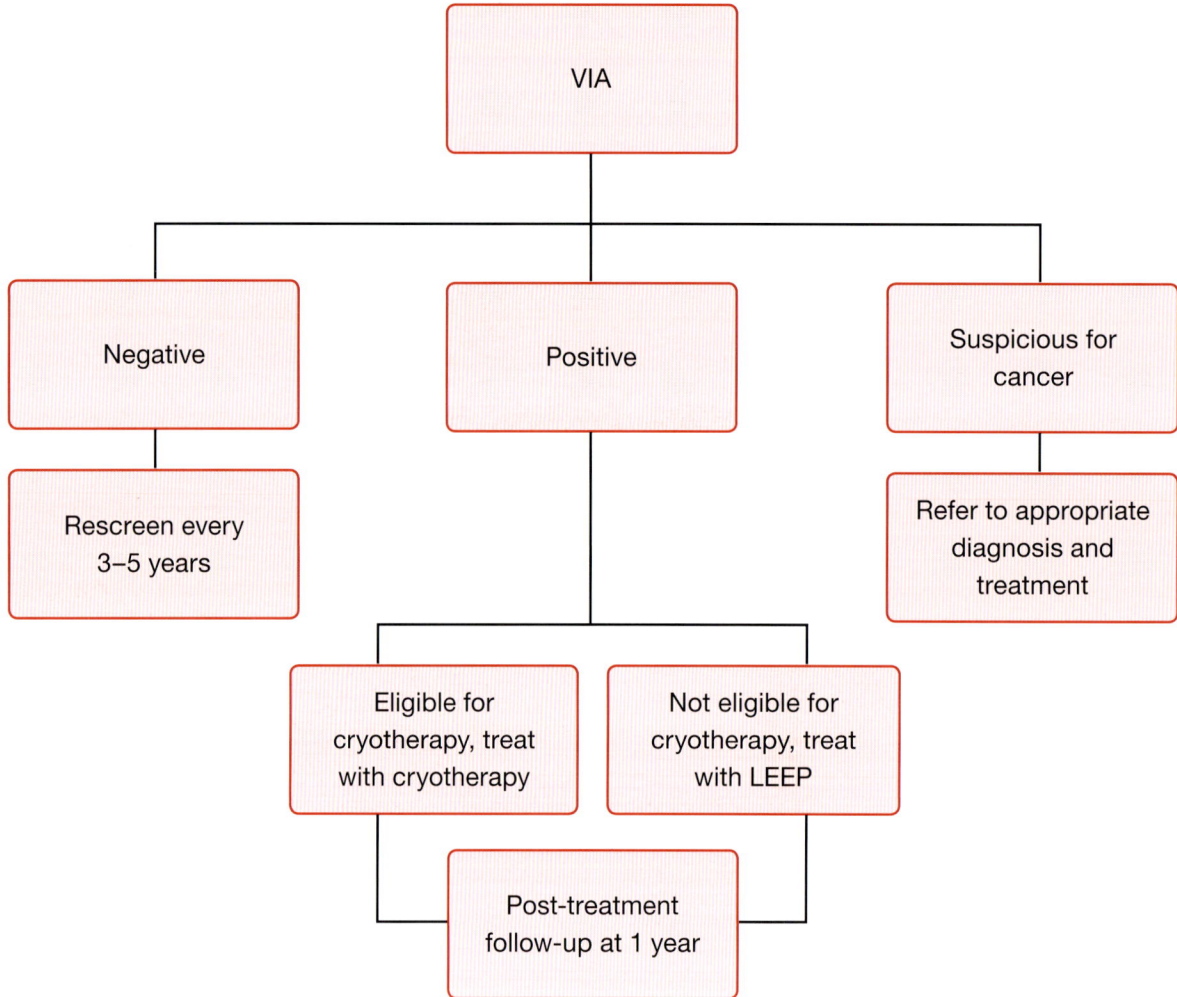

Note: Refer to the screen-and-treat recommendations provided in Chapter 3 of the guideline for guidance about which strategies are recommended, and for information on the specific factors to consider when deciding on a strategy.

Screen with an HPV test followed by colposcopy (with or without biopsy)[1] and treat with cryotherapy, or LEEP when not eligible for cryotherapy

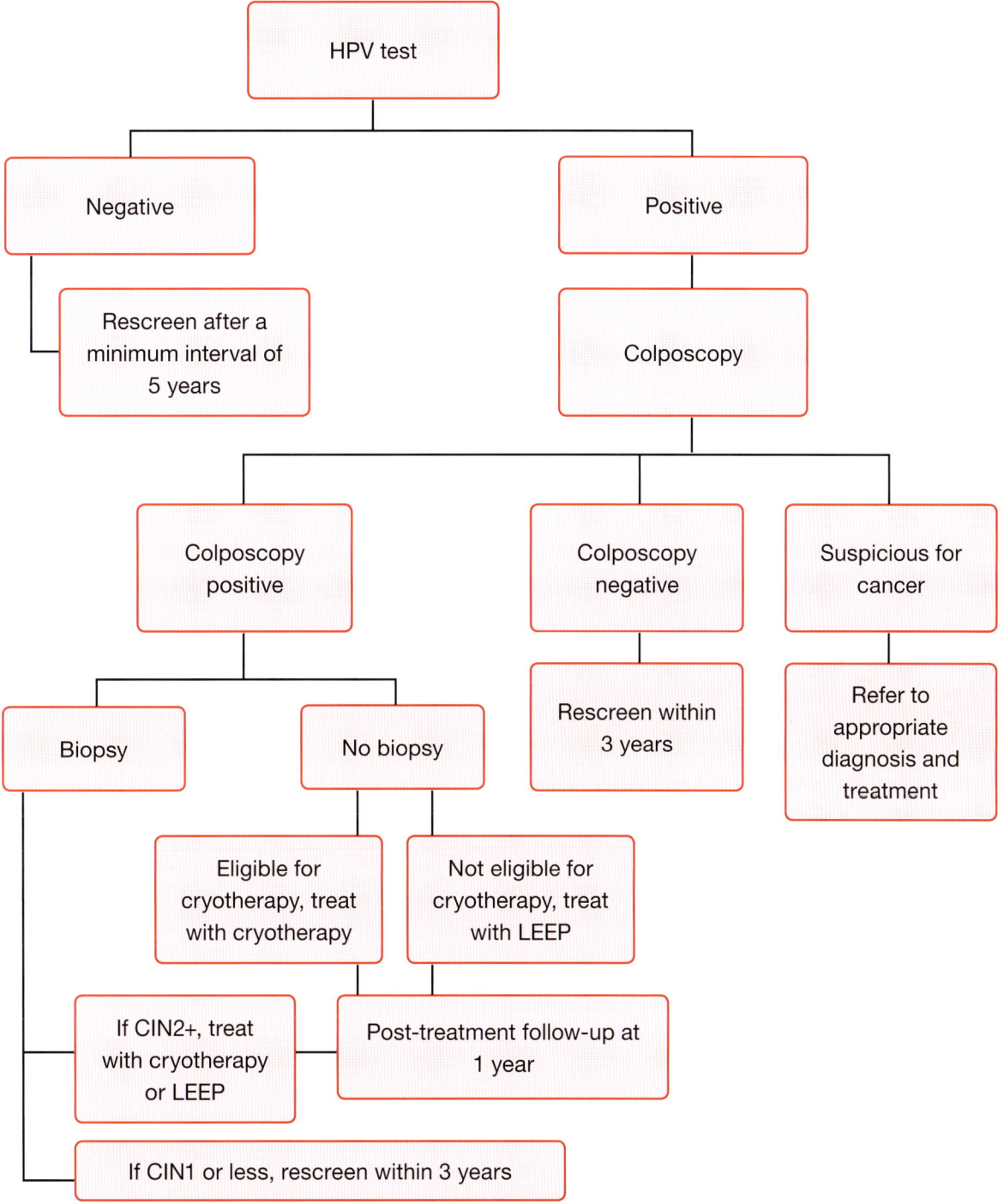

Note: Refer to the screen-and-treat recommendations provided in Chapter 3 of the guideline for guidance about which strategies are recommended, and for information on the specific factors to consider when deciding on a strategy.

---

[1] Women with positive colposcopic impression can receive biopsy for histological confirmation or be treated immediately.

Screen with cytology followed by colposcopy (with or without biopsy)[1] and treat with cryotherapy, or LEEP when not eligible for cryotherapy

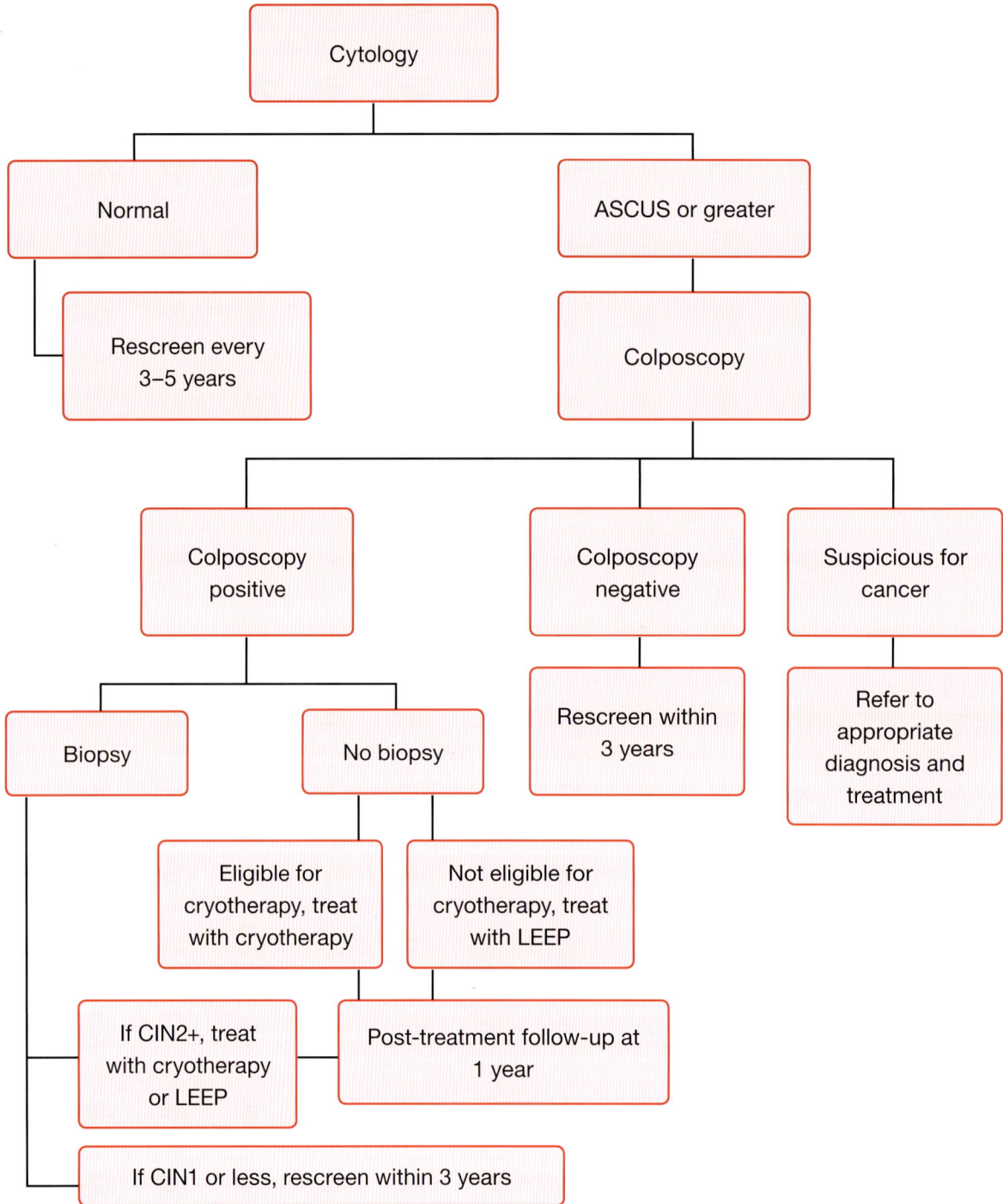

Note: Refer to the screen-and-treat recommendations provided in Chapter 3 of the guideline for guidance about which strategies are recommended, and for information on the specific factors to consider when deciding on a strategy.

---

[1] Women with positive colposcopic impression can receive biopsy for histological confirmation or be treated immediately.

Annex 4. Flowcharts for screen-and-treat strategies (HIV-positive status or unknown HIV status in areas with high endemic HIV infection)

The following flowcharts describe the steps for each of the screen-and-treat strategies that are available. The flowcharts *do not* indicate which strategy is preferred. Refer to the screen-and-treat recommendations provided in Chapter 3 of the guideline for guidance about which strategies are recommended, and to the decision-making flowchart in Annex 2. For detailed information about the specific factors the guideline panel considered when making the recommendations, refer to the evidence-to-recommendation tables for each recommendation (Supplemental material, Sections A and B).

Screen with an HPV test and treat with cryotherapy, or LEEP when not eligible for cryotherapy

When an HPV test is positive, treatment is provided. With this strategy, visual inspection with acetic acid (VIA) is used to determine **eligibility** for cryotherapy.

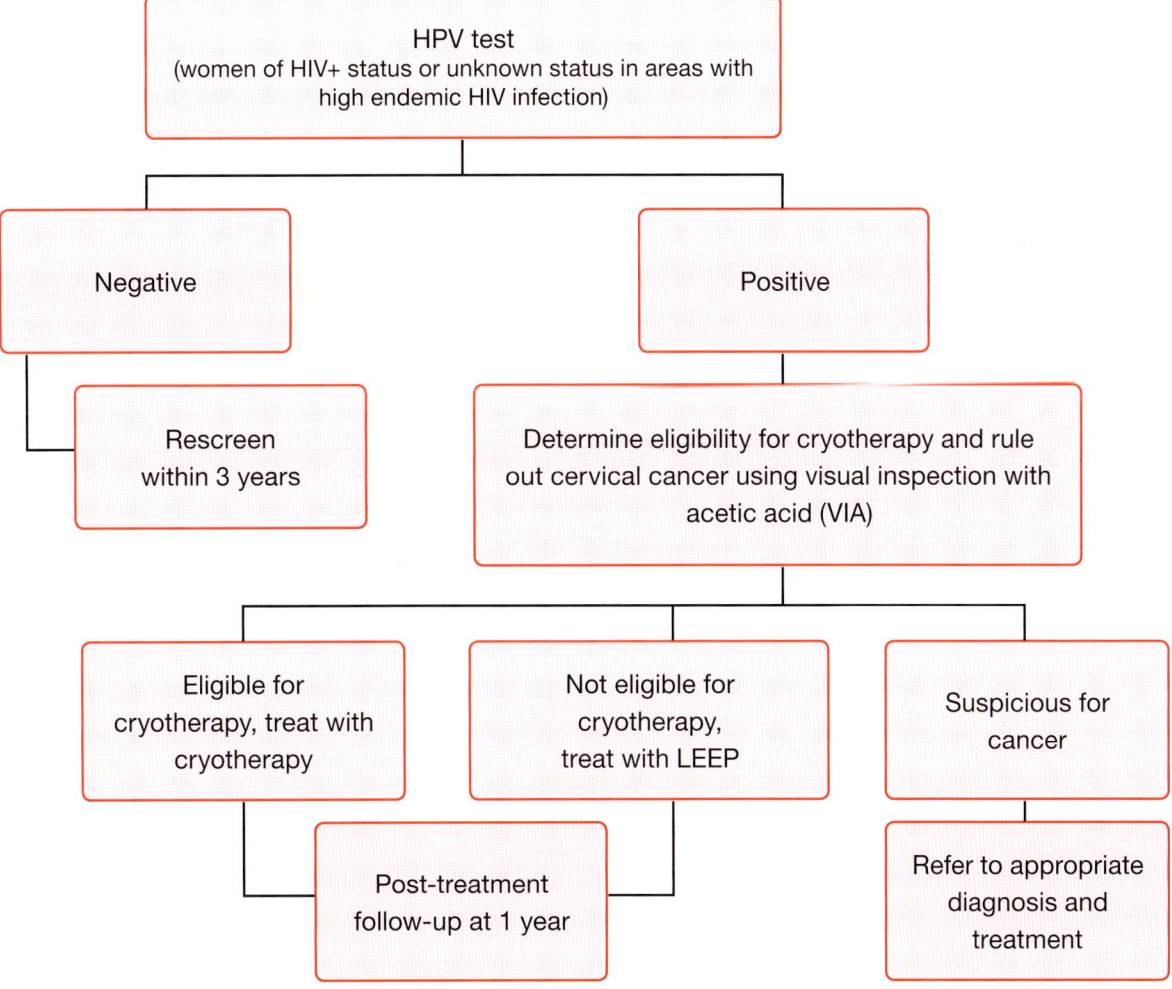

Note: Refer to the screen-and-treat recommendations provided in Chapter 3 of the guideline for guidance about which strategies are recommended, and for information on the factors to consider when deciding on a strategy.

Screen with an HPV test followed by VIA and treat with cryotherapy, or LEEP when not eligible for cryotherapy

When an HPV test is positive, then VIA is provided as a second screening test to determine whether or not treatment is offered. Treatment is only provided if BOTH the HPV test and VIA are positive.

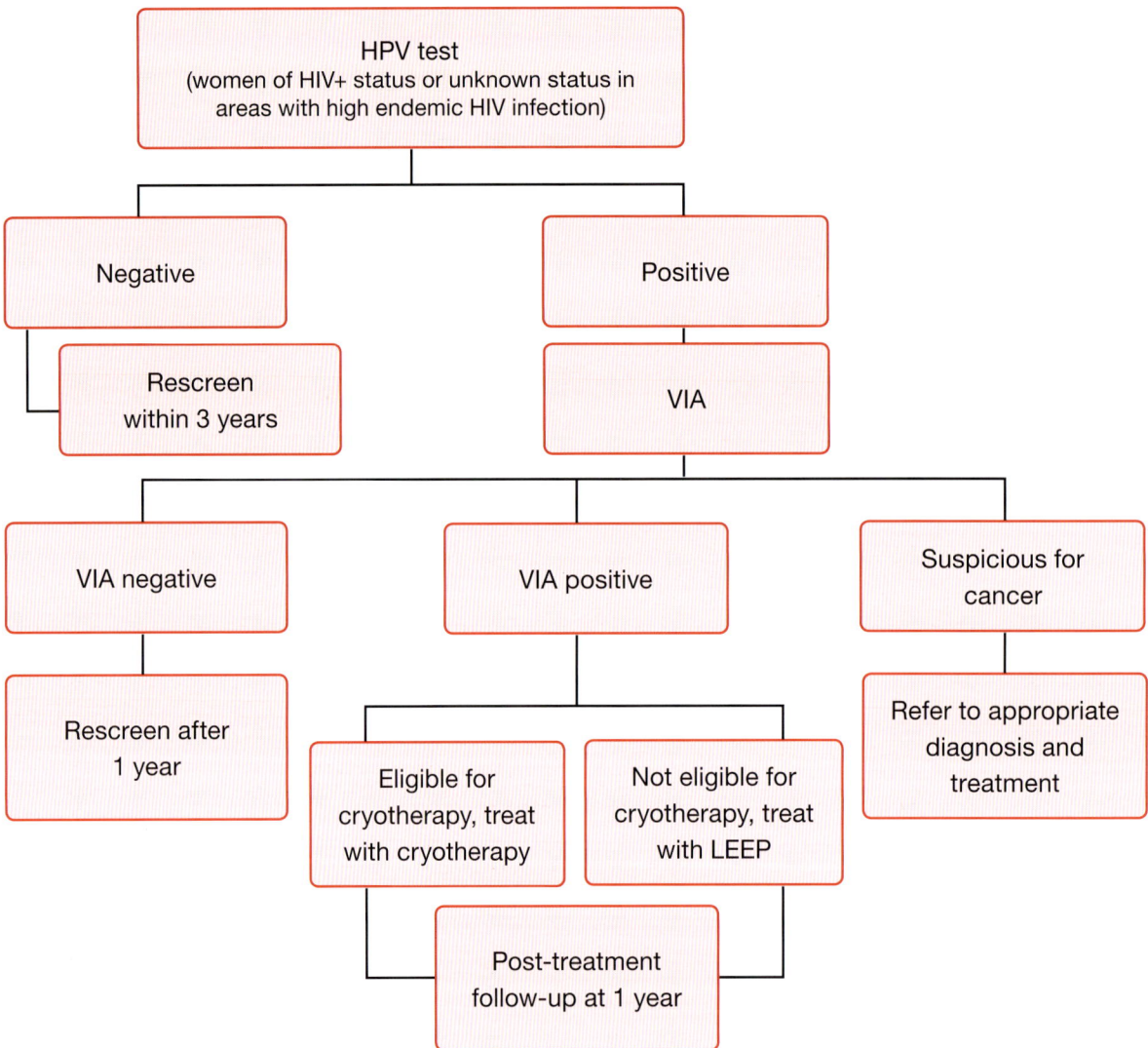

Note: Refer to the screen-and-treat recommendations provided in Chapter 3 of the guideline for guidance about which strategies are recommended, and for information on the factors to consider when deciding on a strategy.

Screen with VIA and treat with cryotherapy, or LEEP when not eligible for cryotherapy

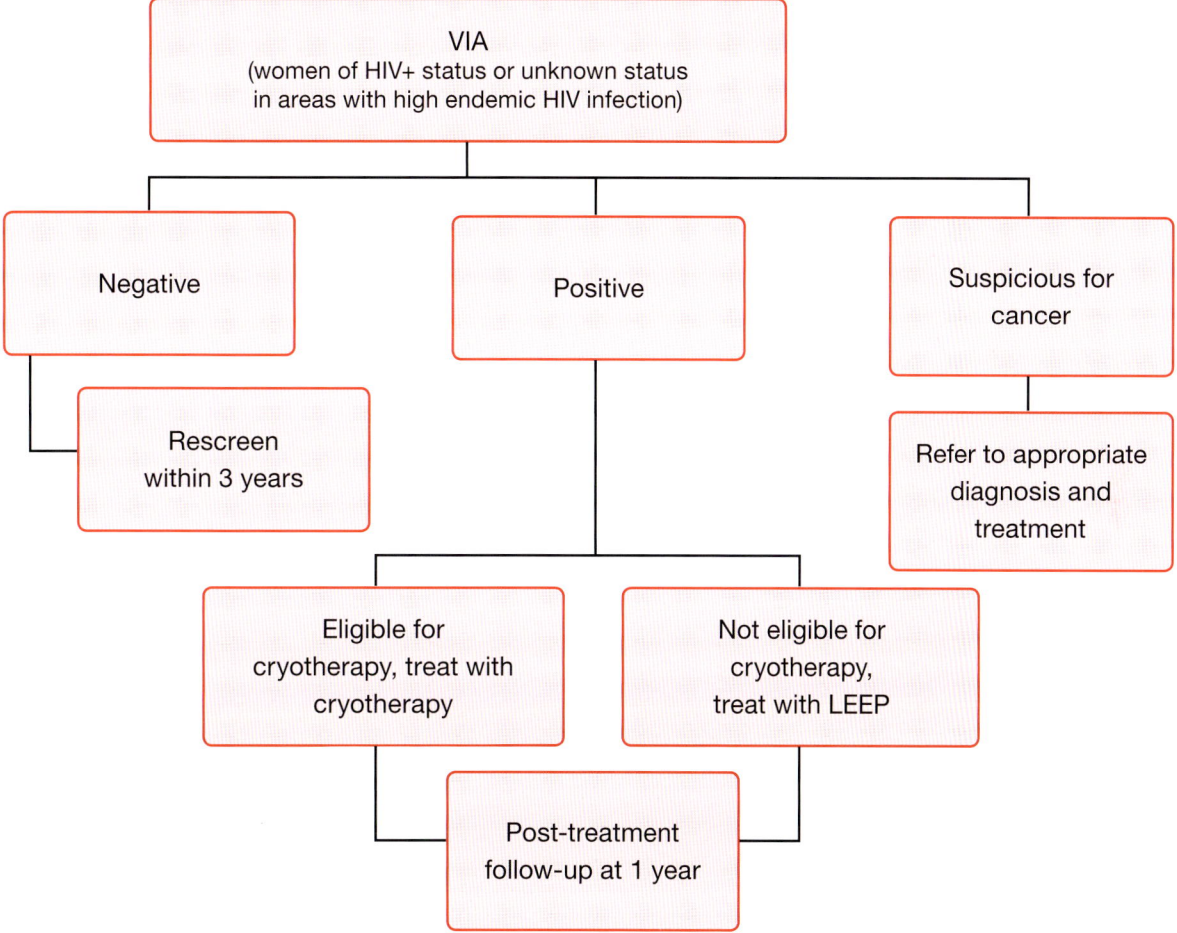

Note: Refer to the screen-and-treat recommendations provided in Chapter 3 of the guideline for guidance about which strategies are recommended, and for information on the factors to consider when deciding on a strategy.

Screen with an HPV test followed by colposcopy (with or without biopsy)[1] and treat with cryotherapy, or LEEP when not eligible for cryotherapy

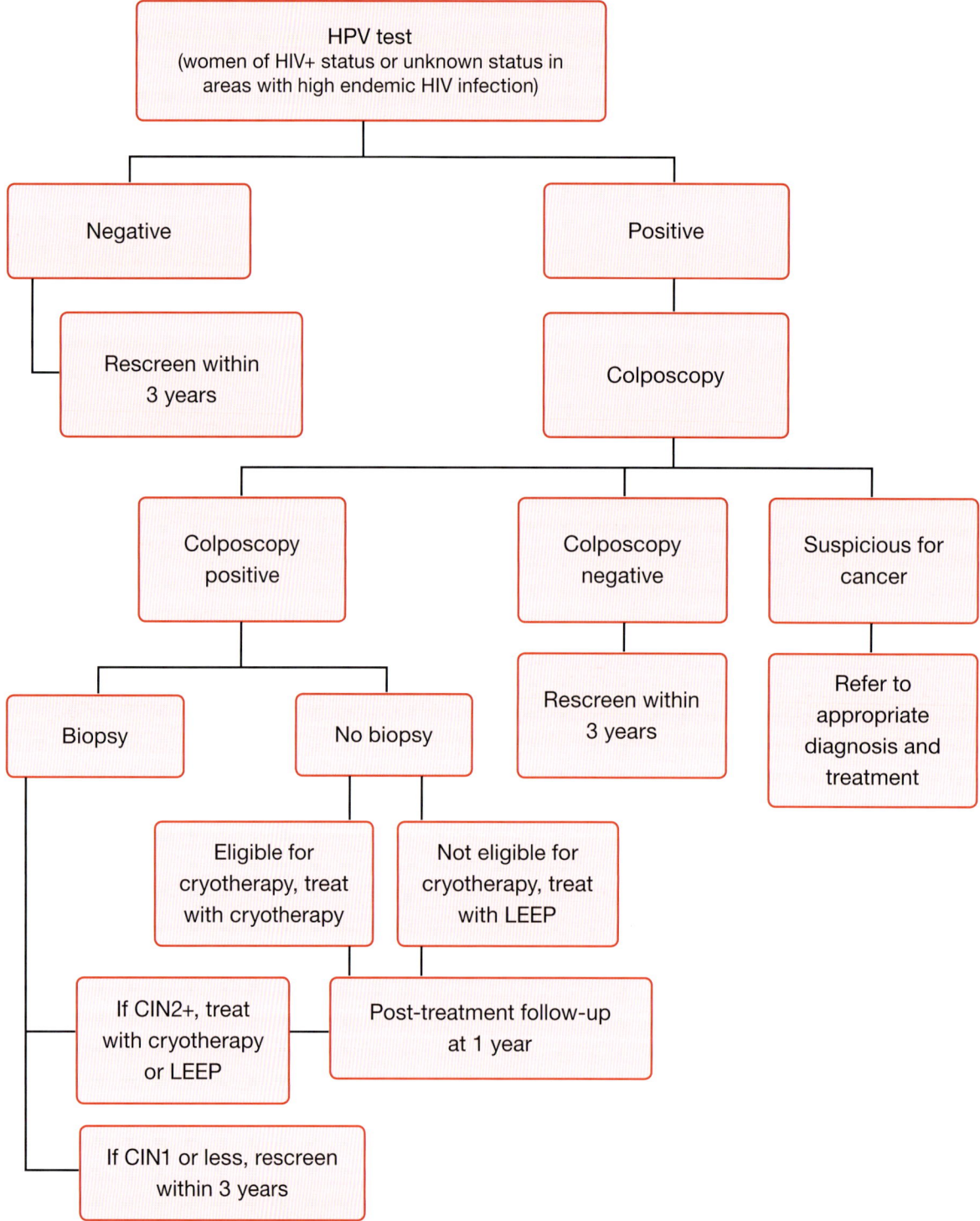

Note: Refer to the screen-and-treat recommendations provided in Chapter 3 of the guideline for guidance about which strategies are recommended, and for information on the factors to consider when deciding on a strategy.

---

[1] Women with positive colposcopic impression can receive biopsy for histological confirmation or be treated immediately.

WHO guidelines for screening and treatment of precancerous lesions for cervical cancer prevention

Screen with cytology followed by colposcopy (with or without biopsy)[1] and treat with cryotherapy or LEEP (when not eligible for cryotherapy)

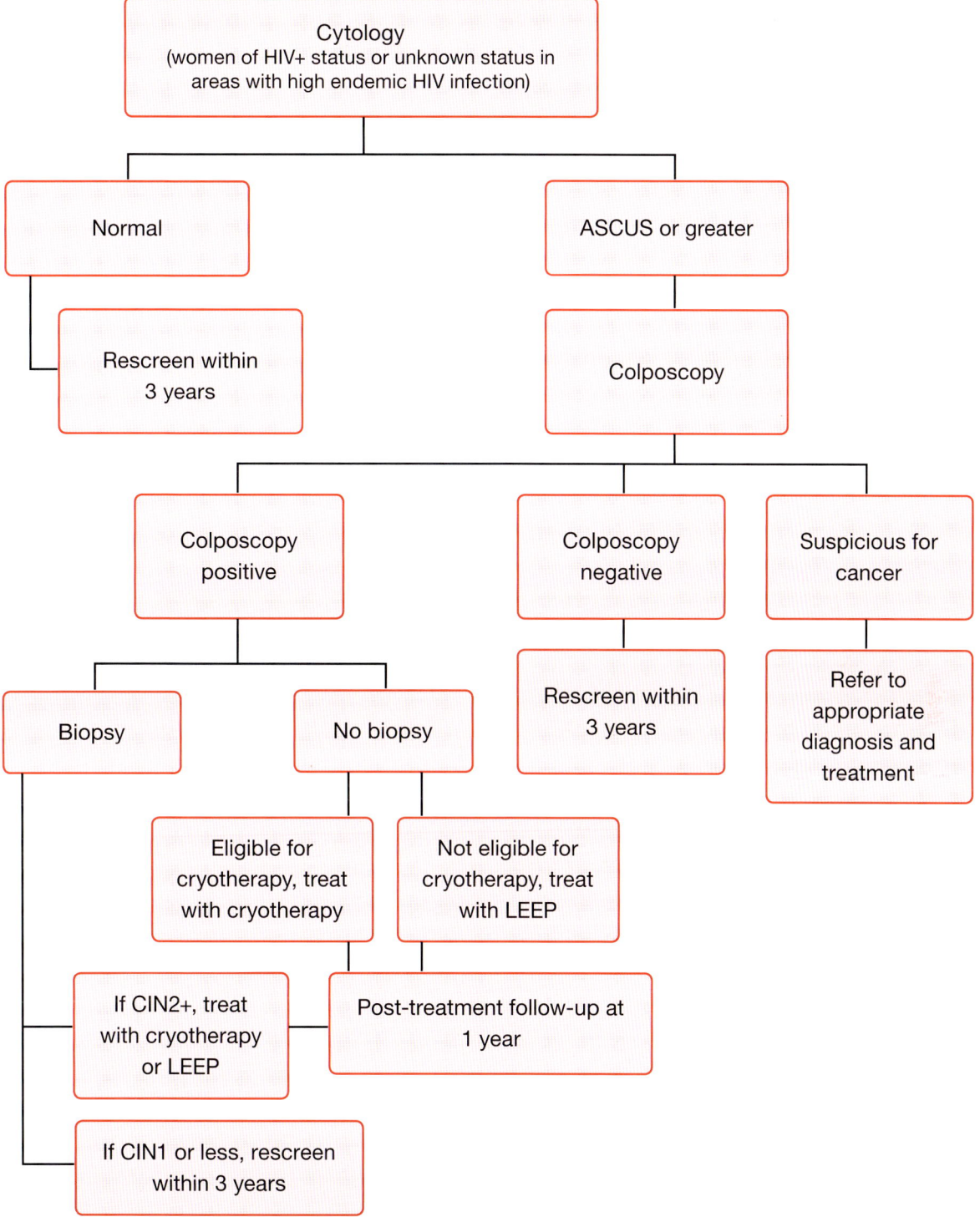

Note: Refer to the screen-and-treat recommendations provided in Chapter 3 of the guideline for guidance about which strategies are recommended, and for information on the factors to consider when deciding on a strategy.

---

[1] Women with positive colposcopic impression can receive biopsy for histological confirmation or be treated immediately.

Annex 5. Search strategies for evidence reviews

Diagnostic test accuracy of HPV (human papillomavirus) testing, VIA (visual inspection with acetic acid), Pap testing (cytology), and colposcopy

VIA compared to other tests:

Search in OVID MEDLINE (up to January 2012)

1. cervical intraepithelial neoplasia/
2. uterine cervical dysplasia/
3. uterine cervical neoplasms/
4. ((precancer* or pre-cancer* or neoplas* or dysplasia or lesion* or premalignan* or malignan* or cancer* or carcinoma*) adj3 cervi*).tw.
5. (cin or cin2* or cin3* or cin1).tw.
6. 1 or 2 or 3 or 4 or 5
7. Acetic Acid/ or acetic acid.tw.
8. (VIA and visual).tw.
9. (visual adj inspection).tw.
10. AAT.tw.
11. or/7-10
12. HPV.tw.
13. (papillomavirus or (papilloma adj virus)).tw.
14. exp papillomaviridae/
15. (or/12-14) and (test* or detect*).tw.
16. Vaginal smears/
17. (pap* adj (smear* or test*)).tw.
18. cytolog*.tw.
19. or/16-18
20. 11 and 15
21. 11 and 19
22. 15 and 19
23. 15 or 20 or 21 or 22
24. 6 and 23
25. sensitiv:.mp.
26. predictive value:.mp.
27. accurac:.tw.
28. screen:.tw.
29. mass screening/
30. diagnostic odds ratio*.tw.
31. likelihood ratio*.tw.
32. (receiver operator characteristic or receiver operating characteristic or receiver operator characteristics or receiver operating characteristics or roc or roc curve).tw.
33. (positiv* adj3 result*).tw.
34. or/25-33
35. 24 and 34

Searches in EMBASE, the Cochrane Library and LILACS

The OVID MEDLINE search was adapted to the subject headings appropriate for each database.

Colposcopy:

Searches in OVID MEDLINE and EMBASE (up to September 2012)

1. exp uterine cervix disease/di
2. cervical intraepithelial neoplasia/
3. uterine cervical dysplasia/
4. uterine cervical neoplasms/
5. ((precancer* or pre-cancer* or neoplas* or dysplasia or lesion* or premalignan* or malignan* or cancer* or carcinoma*) adj3 cervi*).tw.
6. (cin or cin2* or cin3* or cin1).tw.
7. or/1-6
8. (colposcopy and (sensitivity or specificity or receiver operator characteristic or receiver operating characteristic or receiver operator characteristics or receiver operating characteristics or roc or roc curve or predictive value or likelihood ratio or accurac* or diagnosis or diagnostic)).tw.
9. 7 and 8

Annex 6. PRISMA flow diagram for inclusion and exclusion of studies for evidence reviews

Diagnostic test accuracy of HPV (human papillomavirus) testing, VIA (visual inspection with acetic acid), Pap testing (cytology), and colposcopy

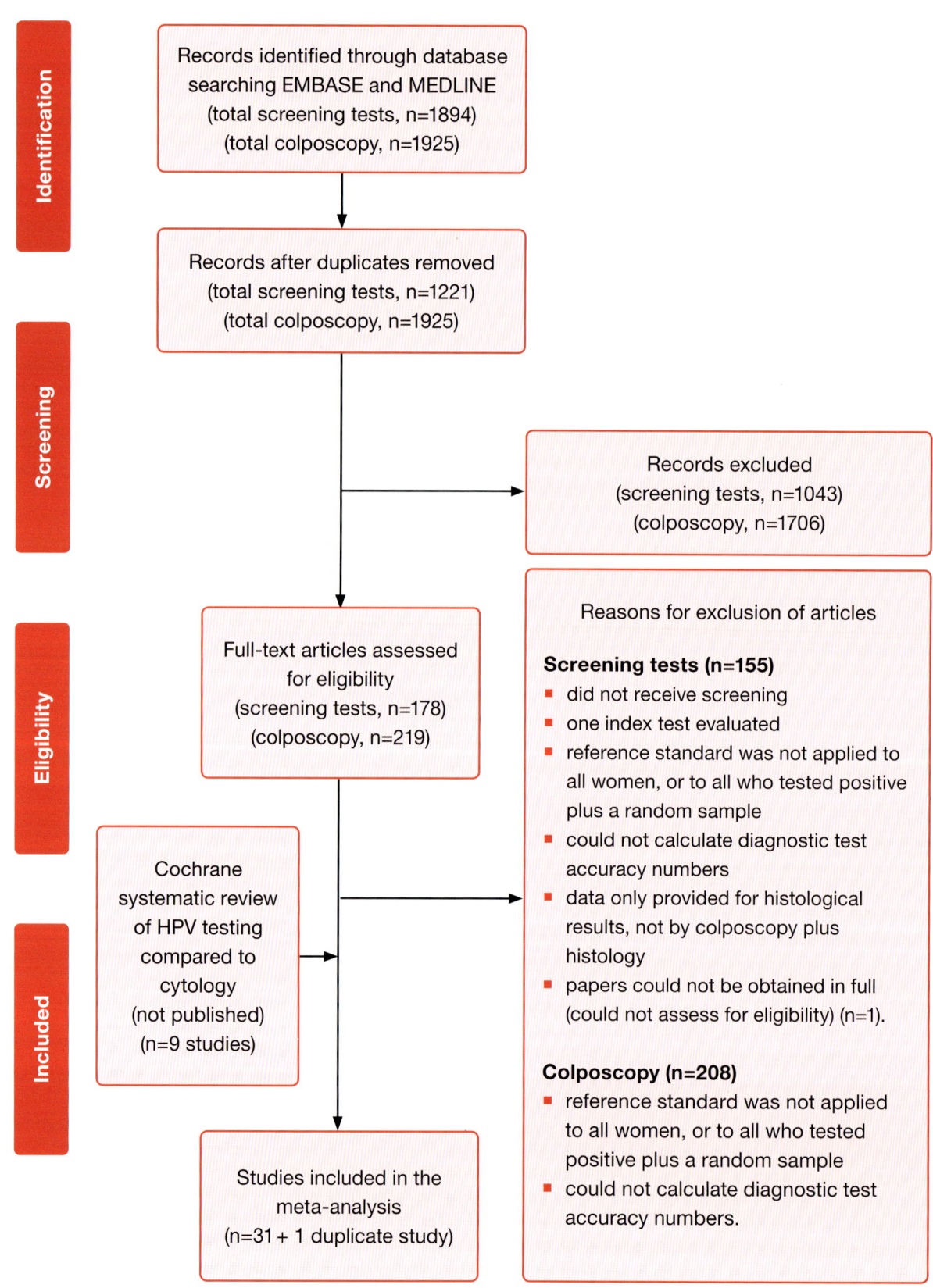

Annex 7. Reference list of all studies included in the evidence reviews

Studies on diagnostic test accuracy

Agorastos T et al. Human papillomavirus testing for primary screening in women at low risk of developing cervical cancer. The Greek experience. *Gynecologic Oncology,* 2005, 96(3):714–720.

Belinson J et al. Shanxi Province Cervical Cancer Screening Study: a cross-sectional comparative trial of multiple techniques to detect cervical neoplasia. *Gynecologic Oncology*, 2001, 83(2):439–444.

Bigras G, De Marval F. The probability for a Pap test to be abnormal is directly proportional to HPV viral load: Results from a Swiss study comparing HPV testing and liquid-based cytology to detect cervical cancer precursors in 13 842 women. *British Journal of Cancer*, 2005, 93(5):575–581.

Cantor SB et al. Accuracy of colposcopy in the diagnostic setting compared with the screening setting. *Obstetrics & Gynecology*, 2008, 111(1):7–14.

Cardenas-Turanzas M et al. The performance of human papillomavirus high-risk DNA testing in the screening and diagnostic settings. *Cancer Epidemiology Biomarkers and Prevention*, 2008, 17(10):2865–2871.

Cremer M et al. Adequacy of visual inspection with acetic acid in women of advancing age. *International Journal of Gynaecology & Obstetrics*, 2011, 113(1):68–71.

Cremer ML et al. Digital assessment of the reproductive tract versus colposcopy for directing biopsies in women with abnormal Pap smears. *Journal of Lower Genital Tract Disease*, 2010, 14(1):5–10.

Cristoforoni PM et al. Computerized colposcopy: results of a pilot study and analysis of its clinical relevance. *Obstetrics & Gynecology*, 1995, 85(6):1011–1016.

de Cremoux P et al. Efficiency of the hybrid capture 2 HPV DNA test in cervical cancer screening. A study by the French Society of Clinical Cytology. *American Journal of Clinical Pathology*, 2003, 120(4):492–499.

Depuydt CE et al. BD-ProExC as adjunct molecular marker for improved detection of CIN2+ after HPV primary screening. *Cancer Epidemiology Biomarkers and Prevention*, 2011, 20(4):628–637.

De Vuyst H et al. Comparison of Pap smear, visual inspection with acetic acid, human papillomavirus DNA-PCR testing and cervicography. *International Journal of Gynecology & Obstetrics*, 2005, 89(2):120–126.

Durdi GS et al. Correlation of colposcopy using Reid colposcopic index with histopathology – a prospective study. *Journal of the Turkish German Gynecology Association*, 2009, 10(4):205–207.

Elit L et al. Assessment of two cervical screening methods in Mongolia: cervical cytology and visual inspection with acetic acid. *Journal of Lower Genital Tract Disease*, 2006, 10(2):83–88.

Ferris DG, Miller MD. Colposcopic accuracy in a residency training program: defining competency and proficiency. *Journal of Family Practice*, 1993, 36(5):515–520.

Ghaemmaghami F et al. Visual inspection with acetic acid as a feasible screening test for cervical neoplasia in Iran. *International Journal of Gynecological Cancer*, 2004, 14(3):465–469.

Goel A et al. Visual inspection of the cervix with acetic acid for cervical intraepithelial lesions. *International Journal of Gynecology & Obstetrics*, 2005, 88(1):25–30.

Hedge D et al. Diagnostic value of acetic acid comparing with conventional Pap smear in the detection of colposcopic biopsy-proved CIN. *Journal of Cancer Research & Therapeutics*, 2011, 7(4):454–458.

Homesley HD, Jobson VW, Reish RL. Use of colposcopically directed, four-quadrant cervical biopsy by the colposcopy trainee. *Journal of Reproductive Medicine*, 1984, 29(5):311–316.

Hovland S et al. A comprehensive evaluation of the accuracy of cervical pre-cancer detection methods in a high-risk area in East Congo. *British Journal of Cancer*, 2010, 102(6):957–965.

Jones DE et al. Evaluation of the atypical Pap smear. *American Journal of Obstetrics & Gynecology*, 1987, 157(3):544–549.

Kierkegaard O et al. Diagnostic accuracy of cytology and colposcopy in cervical squamous intraepithelial lesions. *Acta Obstetricia et Gynecologica Scandinavica*, 1994, 73(8):648–651.

Mahmud SM et al. Comparison of human papillomavirus testing and cytology for cervical cancer screening in a primary health care setting in the Democratic Republic of the Congo. *Gynecologic Oncology*, 2012, 124(2):286–291.

Monsonego J et al. Evaluation of oncogenic human papillomavirus RNA and DNA tests with liquid-based cytology in primary cervical cancer screening: the FASE study. *International Journal of Cancer*, 2011, 129(3):691–701.

Mousavi AS et al. A prospective study to evaluate the correlation between Reid colposcopic index impression and biopsy histology. *Journal of Lower Genital Tract Disease*, 2007, 11(3):147–150.

Pan Q et al. A thin-layer, liquid-based Pap test for mass screening in an area of China with a high incidence of cervical carcinoma a cross-sectional, comparative study. *Acta Cytologica*, 2003, 47(1):45–50.

Patil K et al. Comparison of diagnostic efficacy of visual inspection of cervix with acetic acid and Pap smear for prevention of cervical cancer: is VIA superseding Pap smear? *Journal of SAFOG*, 2011, 3(3):131–134.

Petry KU et al. Inclusion of HPV testing in routine cervical cancer screening for women above 29 years in Germany: results for 8466 patients. *British Journal of Cancer*, 2003, 88(10):1570–1577.

Qiao YL et al. A new HPV-DNA test for cervical-cancer screening in developing regions: a cross-sectional study of clinical accuracy in rural China. *Lancet Oncology*, 2008, 9(10):929–936.

Sahasrabuddhe VV et al. Comparison of visual inspection with acetic acid and cervical cytology to detect high-grade cervical neoplasia among HIV-infected women in India. *International Journal of Cancer*, 2012, 130(1):234–240.

Sankaranarayanan R et al. Test characteristics of visual inspection with 4% acetic acid (VIA) and Lugol's iodine (VILI) in cervical cancer screening in Kerala, India. *International Journal of Cancer*, 2003, 106(3):404–408.

Shastri SS et al. Concurrent evaluation of visual, cytological and HPV testing as screening methods for the early detection of cervical neoplasia in Mumbai, India. *Bulletin of the World Health Organization*, 2005, 83(3):186–194.

Sodhani P et al. Test characteristics of various screening modalities for cervical cancer: a feasibility study to develop an alternative strategy for resource-limited settings. *Cytopathology*, 2006, 17(6):348–352.

Studies on baseline risks included in the model

Arbyn M et al. Evidence regarding human papillomavirus testing in secondary prevention of cervical cancer. *Vaccine*, 2012, 30 Suppl 5:F88–99.

Denny L et al. Human papillomavirus infection and cervical disease in human immunodeficiency virus-1-infected women. *Obstetrics & Gynecology*, 2008, 111(6):1380–1387.

De Vuyst H et al. HIV, human papillomavirus, and cervical neoplasia and cancer in the era of highly active antiretroviral therapy. *European Journal of Cancer Prevention*, 2008, 17(6):545–554.

De Vuyst H et al. Prevalence and determinants of human papillomavirus infection and cervical lesions in HIV-positive women in Kenya. *British Journal of Cancer*, 2012, 107(9):1624–1630.

GLOBOCAN 2008 [online database]. France, World Health Organization, International Agency for Research on Cancer, 2010 (http://globocan.iarc.fr/, accessed 15 August 2013).

Joshi S et al. Screening of cervical neoplasia in HIV-infected women in India. *AIDS*, 2013, 27(4):607–615.

Sankaranarayanan R et al; Osmanabad District Cervical Screening Study Group. A cluster randomized controlled trial of visual, cytology and human papillomavirus screening for cancer of the cervix in rural India. *International Journal of Cancer*, 2005, 116(4):617–623.

Zhang HY et al. HPV prevalence and cervical intraepithelial neoplasia among HIV-infected women in Yunnan Province, China: a pilot study. *Asian Pacific Journal of Cancer Prevention*, 2012, 13(1):91–96.